ARTHROSCOPIC SURGERY

ARTHROSCOPIC SURGERY

THE WRIST

Terry L. Whipple, M.D.
Orthopaedic Research of Virginia
Tuckahoe Orthopaedic Associates
Richmond, Virginia

Clinical Professor of Orthopaedics
The Bowman Gray School of Medicine
Wake Forest University
Winston-Salem, North Carolina

Illustrated by Susan E. Brust, M.S.

With 1 Contributor

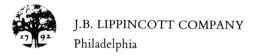

J.B. LIPPINCOTT COMPANY
Philadelphia

Associate Editor: Delois Patterson
Project Editor: Molly E. Dickmeyer
Indexer: Ann Cassar
Designer: Doug Smock
Cover Designer: Tom Jackson
Production Manager: Caren Erlichman
Production Coordinator: Sharon McCarthy
Compositor: Tapsco Incorporated
Printer/Binder: R. R. Donnelley and Sons
Color Printer: Lehigh Colortronics

6   5   4   3   2   1

Library of Congress Cataloging-in-Publication Data

Whipple, Terry L.
    Arthroscopic surgery—the wrist / Terry L. Whipple.
        p.   cm.
    Includes bibliographical references and index.
    ISBN 0-397-51023-3: $150.00
    1. Wrist—Endoscopic surgery.   I. Title.
    RD559.W45   1992
    617.5′74—dc20   91-32560
                                                                                  CIP

The authors and publisher have exerted every effort to ensure that drug selection and dosage set forth in this text are in accord with current recommendations and practice at the time of publication. However, in view of ongoing research, changes in government regulations, and the constant flow of information relating to drug therapy and drug reactions, the reader is urged to check the package insert for each drug for any change in indications and dosage and for added warnings and precautions. This is particularly important when the recommended agent is a new or infrequently employed drug.

Dedication

To my wife, Lynda, and to Ryan, Haley, Scott, and Keith

CONTRIBUTOR

James C. Y. Chow, M.D.
Private Practice
Mount Vernon, Illinois

Clinical Assistant Professor
Southern Illinois University
School of Medicine
Springfield, Illinois

FOREWORD

Arthroscopy has inaugurated a new era in orthopaedic surgery by providing the technical capability to directly examine pathology within various joints. Arthroscopy of the wrist has the potential to redefine the nature of intra-articular injuries to this complex joint, and also to facilitate definitive treatment for many common pathologic conditions. The efficiency of arthroscopy in determining the size, extent, and location of tears of the triangular fibrocartilage and the degree of injury to scapholunate and lunotriquetral ligaments is widely recognized. The articular surface of the distal radius can be examined for areas of cartilage damage associated with fractures, and articular fracture fragments can be better aligned with the aid of this minimally invasive procedure. Examination of the radiocarpal and midcarpal joints permits more thorough evaluation of carpal instabilities.

When analyzing the indications and techniques for a new procedure such as wrist arthroscopy, nothing serves the orthopaedic surgeon better than a single source on which to rely for judgement and operative skills. In *Arthroscopic Surgery: The Wrist,* the author presents the basic requirements of patient history and physical examination, diagnostic testing, and radiographic imaging of the wrist. The required instrumentation, surgical-suite preparations, and intraoperative set-up for wrist arthroscopy are clearly and concisely defined. The text beautifully illustrates pertinent intraarticular and extraarticular surgical anatomy as an aid to the novice as well as the experienced arthroscopist or hand surgeon. The author particularly emphasizes relevant functional anatomy, which helps to reinforce the fine points of operative procedures. Potential obstacles are addressed in detail to ensure that wrist arthroscopy can be performed safely and successfully.

After discussion of appropriate surgical environment and guides to proper diagnostic arthroscopic techniques, the book addresses specific pathologic conditions affecting the wrist. Not only are the diagnostic benefits of arthroscopy emphasized, but appropriate therapeutic procedures for specific disorders are also described so a clear approach to definitive treatment can be followed. Discussion of complications related to the technique and methods to avoid pitfalls and problems assist the arthroscopic surgeon in developing an efficient program for smooth and comprehensive evaluation and treatment of patients with wrist disorders.

On behalf of those with a keen interest in arthroscopy of the wrist, we cannot thank Dr. Whipple enough for his innovative developments and perfection of this important addition to the surgeon's diagnostic and surgical armamentarium. Clearly no one has worked harder to define the role of arthroscopy in diagnosis and potential treatment of disorders of the wrist than the author of this text. We as arthroscopic surgeons are most grateful for his untiring efforts to present these new techniques through instructional courses, laboratory seminars, demonstrations, and publications. From the time of the first wrist arthroscopy workshop at Bowman Gray School of Medicine in 1986, Dr. Whipple has been a leading contributor to the advancement of wrist arthroscopy. Students of the wrist and all surgeons who wish to expand their operative skills and develop significant expertise in this exciting, advancing specialty of arthroscopic surgery appreciate the outstanding achievements of the physicians who have devoted immeasurable time and energy to its development. *Surgical Arthroscopy: The Wrist* consolidates the past endeavors of many clinicians and appropriately applies these techniques to the field of hand and wrist surgery. Further advances will undoubtedly be made, but, for the interested surgeon, there is no better source of direction for a fruitful and gratifying experience with arthroscopy of the wrist than this text.

William P. Cooney, III, M.D.
Professor of Orthopaedic Surgery,
Mayo Medical School,
Head, Section of Hand Surgery,
Mayo Clinic
Rochester, Minnesota

PREFACE

*T*he development of new technology and surgical techniques increase the ability of physicians to provide more effective treatment for their patients. New developments must gain appropriate clinical application with accurate delineation of indications and definition of risk factors before they are widely used. Information must be disseminated adequately to allow surgeons to develop technical expertise with newer methods. This process can be extremely slow at times. This has not been the case, however, with the development and widespread application of wrist arthroscopy.

Immediately following the report of the techniques developed to provide predictable arthroscopic access to the wrist in 1986,[1] there were constant inquiries from surgeons seeking opportunities to learn how to perform wrist arthroscopy effectively and safely. Intense interest was expressed in better methods for evaluating and treating intraarticular pathology in the wrist, which is the most complex joint in human anatomy. Numerous courses were staged in the ensuing months to discuss and teach these techniques, and all of them were oversubscribed. This led to requests for a textbook on the subject, an undertaking that I resisted for four years until refinements in technique and follow-up on clinical experience were sufficient to place in writing recommendations that would be durable and worthy of preservation in textbook format.

I have attempted to develop this text as a reference work for clinical and surgical technique. It is organized from a surgeon's clinical perspective, considering plausible and efficient approaches to a patient who presents with certain constellations of symptoms and signs. Part I considers general approaches to wrist arthroscopy in the context of the patient's clinical presentation. Part II is organized as a reference for minimally invasive surgical approaches to patients with an established diagnosis.

1. *Whipple TL, Marotta JJ, Powell JH III. Techniques of wrist arthroscopy. Journal of Arthroscopy and Related Surgery 1986;2:244.*

Liberal use of illustrations has been made to graphically demonstrate points made in the text. It is my hope that this format will facilitate successful application of techniques for arthroscopic surgery of the wrist when the clinical situation warrants surgical intervention.

—*T.L.W.*

ACKNOWLEDGMENTS

I would like to acknowledge the invaluable professional skills of Susan Brust, who has illustrated this text single-handedly and so effectively. Her co-operation and diligence have brought a consistency of style to the graphic expression of the written text. I am indebted to Connie Lacy for her tireless secretarial efforts in preparation of the manuscript. Chris Wheeler has provided technical assistance with photography and enhancement of arthroscopic images. Judy Cooper, R.N., Frank Ellis, M.D., and Pamela Dillon, my clinical and research team, have been exceptional resources in gathering the information and materials that have gone into this volume. I thank them all sincerely.

CONTENTS

ARTHROSCOPIC SURGERY

Introduction

Arthroscopy has revolutionized the practice of orthopaedic surgery since the mid-1970s. After a long history of sporadic attempts at arthroscopy, technological breakthroughs in Japan and several surgical pioneers in North America launched widespread interest in percutaneous joint surgery.

In 1918, Takagi initiated efforts at endoscopic examination of cadaver knees at the University of Tokyo, using a number 22 French Cystoscope.[1] Bircher advanced the technique in 1921 by using gaseous distention of the knee.[2] In the United States, Kreuscher reported clinical results in diagnostic knee arthroscopy for meniscus disorders in 1925.[3] The large diameter of the cystoscope limited its utility, but in 1931 Takagi developed an arthroscope 3.5 mm in diameter that incorporated a lamp and magnifying optics and provided a clearer visual field. With this device, he compiled unprecedented clinical experience in endoscopic examination of the knee.

In New York, Burman made significant arthroscopic advances. In 1931, he reported using a scope of his own design to examine 100 cadaver knee joints, but he extended his examinations to 25 shoulders, 20 hips, 15 elbows, 3 ankles, and 6 wrists.[4] His arthroscope, used also by colleagues Finkelstein and Mayer in clinical applications, incorporated channels for fluid or gas distention of the joint.[5]

Arthroscopy of the knee was elegantly and convincingly demonstrated by endoscopic photography in Watanabe's *Atlas of Arthroscopy,* published in 1969.[1] Only then did the technique begin to gain clinical credibility and acceptance. Watanabe was a protege of Takagi at the University of Tokyo. He attracted the attention and enthusiasm of several North American surgeons—notably S. Ward Casscells of Wilmington, Delaware; Robert W. Jackson of Toronto, Canada; John Joyce of Philadelphia, Pennsylvania; and Richard O'Connor of West Covina, California. Using the improved Watanabe No. 21 arthroscope with an incandescent bulb at the tip, these surgeons established the application of Watanabe's techniques for knee arthroscopy in the United States and Canada. In various publications, they reported their experience with the numerous advantages of arthroscopy for diagnostic purposes, as well as for early arthroscopic surgery in the knee.[6–10]

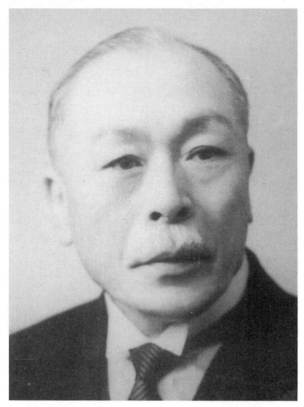

Professor Takagi, Tokyo, Japan

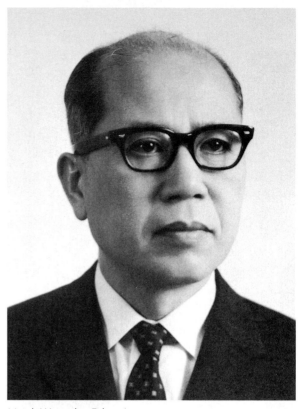

Masaki Watanabe, Tokyo, Japan

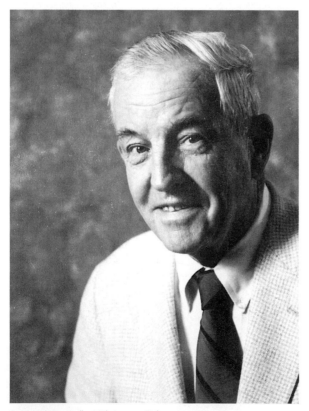

S. Ward Casscells, Wilmington, Delaware

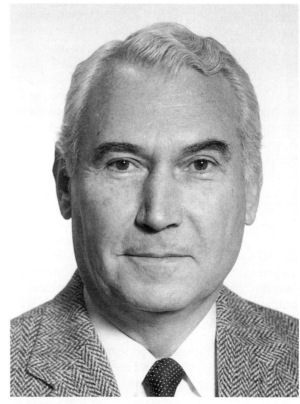

Robert W. Jackson, Toronto, Ontario, Canada

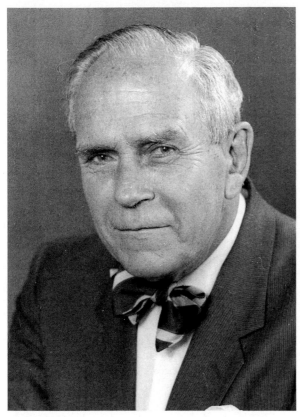

John J. Joyce, III, Philadelphia, Pennsylvania

control heralded a new era in orthopaedics. Minimally invasive surgical techniques have been responsible for earlier definitive treatment of many joint disorders, with the additional advantages of reduced cost and faster recuperation.

Arthroscopy has become an integral part of modern orthopaedic surgery. However, innovative arthroscopic procedures can be most successfully employed when practiced with a firm understanding of their subtle refinements, their limitations, and their risks. This text was inspired by the need for a comprehensive discourse on arthroscopy that is of practical clinical value. It should be a tribute to those pioneering surgeons who dared to do things a little bit differently . . . a little bit better.

REFERENCES

1. Watanabe M, Takeda S, Ikeuchi H. Atlas of arthroscopy. 2nd ed. Tokyo: Igakui-Shoin, 1969.
2. Bircher E. Die Arthroendoskopie. Zentralbl Chir 1921;14:1460.
3. Kreuscher PH. Semilunar cartilage disease, a plan for early recognition by means of the arthroscope and early treatment of this condition. Illinois Medical Journal 1925;47:290.
4. Burman MS. Arthroscopy, a direct visualization of joints: an experimental cadaver study. J Bone Joint Surg [Am] 1931;13(4):669.
5. Finkelstein H, Mayer L. The arthroscope, a new method of examining joints. J Bone Joint Surg [Am] 1931;13:583.
6. Joyce JJ III. History of arthroscopy. In: O'Connor RL, ed. Arthroscopy. Kalamazoo: Upjohn, 1977:11.
7. Casscells SW. Arthroscopy of the knee joint, a review of 150 cases. J Bone Joint Surg [Am] 1971;53:287.
8. Jackson RW, Abe I. The role of arthroscopy in the management of disorders of the knee: an analysis of 200 consecutive examinations. J Bone Joint Surg [Br] 1972;54:310.
9. O'Connor RL. The arthroscope in the management of crystal-induced synovitis of the knee. J Bone Joint Surg [Am] 1973;55:1443.
10. O'Connor RL. Arthroscopy in the diagnosis and treatment of acute ligament injuries of the knee. J Bone Joint Surg [Am] 1974;56(2):333.
11. Watanabe M, Bechtol RC, Nottage WM. History of arthroscopic surgery. In: Shahriaree H, ed. O'Connor textbook of arthroscopic surgery. Philadelphia: JB Lippincott, 1984:1.

The success of increasing numbers of surgeons with arthroscopic procedures inspired John Joyce to organize the International Arthroscopy Association in 1974 at a meeting in Philadelphia. The development of fiberoptic technology led to further improvement in arthroscope designs, providing better illumination and more durable instruments. O'Connor began to devise surgical techniques for the knee through an operating arthroscope that incorporated a channel for accessory instruments.[11] In the decade that followed, hundreds of orthopaedic surgeons around the world assimilated arthroscopy into their routine practices. Power instruments and miniaturized closed-circuit television cameras were developed for use in arthroscopic surgery.

Other joints began to be exposed by the magnification and illumination provided by arthroscopy. The improved precision and reduced morbidity of surgical procedures performed under arthroscopic

The Basics of Wrist Arthroscopy

1

Historical Developments

*I*nterest in arthroscopy of the wrist has developed following successful clinical experience with arthroscopy of the knee, shoulder, elbow, and ankle. The rapid rise in popularity of arthroscopy is due to the limitations of other diagnostic measures for soft-tissue disorders of the wrist. As with other joints, arthroscopic surgical procedures for the wrist offer reduced treatment morbidity, faster recuperation, and earlier return to function than conventional open surgical procedures. The increasing number of indications for wrist arthroscopy reflects a rapid series of developments in surgical instrument technology and a better understanding of wrist mechanics and pathomechanics.

In 1939, Takagi described six arthroscopic procedures in joints other than the knee: four hip procedures, one shoulder procedure, and one ankle procedure; however, none were performed on wrists.[1] Takagi worked extensively on instrument design and developed the No. 11 arthroscope with a diameter of 2.7 mm. This instrument was small enough for wrist applications, but did not produce a well-focused image. In 1968, Nippon Sheet Glass Company of Osaka, Japan, and Nippon Electric Company of Tokyo, Japan jointly developed a new glass material for the transmission of laser beams. This material, Selfoc (a trade name meaning "self-focusing"), produced lenses that had a very wide range of focus, permitting clear visualization of objects within 1 mm of the lens. Watanabe incorporated this lens material into new arthroscope designs in 1970, ultimately producing a 1.7-mm instrument with a 55° to 70° viewing angle.[2] With this No. 24 arthroscope, Watanabe examined numerous smaller joints between 1970 and 1972, including 21 wrists. This was the earliest reported experience with wrist arthroscopy.

The confined space between articular surfaces and the numerous vulnerable tendons, nerves, and vessels overlying the wrist joint made percutaneous access to the wrist difficult. Subsequent sporadic attempts at arthroscopy of the wrist were compromised by the small visual field provided by the earlier arthroscopes. In 1985, Whipple and Powell conducted a series of cadaver studies to develop a predictable and coordinated system of portals for arthroscopic access to the radiocarpal and midcarpal spaces and to the distal radioulnar joint (DRUJ).[3] Wide-angle lenses were produced for 1.9-mm and 2.7-mm arthroscopes to provide a 90° field of view. Subsequently, 25° and 70° prisms were developed for these scopes to permit offset viewing. As a result of these studies and developments, reliable techniques for arthroscopic examination of the wrist were defined.

Whipple undertook successful clinical trials of wrist arthroscopy in 1985. The interval between the third and fourth extensor compartments was used as the primary access to the radiocarpal space, and the interval between the extensor carpi radialis brevis (ECRB) and index extensor digitorum communis (EDC) tendons provided access to the midcarpal space. Good visualization was achieved without injury to structures overlying the joint. Joint distraction was used to enlarge the intraarticular spaces.

Encouraged by Whipple's initial clinical experience, Poehling used the newly developed techniques and corroborated their safety and efficacy. Wrist arthroscopy has since gained widespread acceptance. The ability to view internal anatomy and pathologic changes without disrupting the supporting capsule and ligamentous structures of the wrist has enabled earlier and more accurate diagnoses of certain wrist disorders and has contributed to a better understanding of wrist mechanics.

INDICATIONS

Wrist arthroscopy is a valuable adjunct to the diagnosis of certain wrist joint problems, and the indications for this procedure continue to increase. It has proven valuable in three general circumstances: intraarticular soft-tissue disorders, intraarticular fractures, and symptomatic wrists with unconfirmed diagnoses. As will be discussed in subsequent chapters, soft-tissue disorders of the wrist are legion and are often difficult to identify precisely. Adjunct imaging techniques such as arthrography, isotope scans, and magnetic resonance imaging are helpful, but are not always sufficient to establish exact diagnoses. Arthroscopic examination may then provide additional identification or qualification of intraarticular pathology.

For patients with arthrograms indicating ex-travasation of dye from the radiocarpal or midcarpal space or the DRUJ, arthroscopy can be used to assess the size and precise location of the ligament or cartilage defect. Better delineation of intraarticular lesions aids in planning appropriate corrective treatment. For patients with carpal instability, wrist arthroscopy can be used to assess the integrity of articular surfaces when contemplating an appropriate stabilizing procedure. For individuals allergic to contrast medium or for whom arthrography is contraindicated, arthroscopic examination provides a highly sensitive and specific means of diagnosing tears of the triangular fibrocartilage (TFC) or disruption of the intrinsic ligaments of the wrist. Arthroscopic access also provides a minimally invasive and relatively atraumatic means of obtaining biopsies of synovial tissue for diagnosis or for performing intraarticular synovectomy in cases of chronic synovial hypertrophy.

Intraarticular fractures are best treated by accurate reduction and restoration of the normal contours of articular surfaces. Arthroscopic visualization is an extremely useful means of monitoring accurate reduction of articular fracture fragments of the distal radius, including displaced die-punch fractures in which portions of the lunate facet of the radius are depressed. Associated fracture debris and fibrin clots can be cleared from the joint at the same time. In addition, certain fractures of the scaphoid can be accurately reduced and stabilized under arthroscopic control without damaging adjacent articular surfaces.

More commonly, wrist arthroscopy is useful for patients with persistent symptoms when other imaging techniques and diagnostic modalities have been inconclusive. When clinical findings are not consistent with subjective complaints, arthroscopic examination may help to identify the presence of occult intraarticular pathology or confirm its absence. Even when conventional work-up establishes an accurate diagnosis, the definitive treatment may carry a high risk of morbidity or complications. In this situation, arthroscopic examination may further define the extent of the pathology and the necessity or urgency for definitive procedures.

Despite the advantages of direct visual examination of the wrist joint, arthroscopy should not preempt conservative management or other conventional techniques for diagnosis of wrist pathology. It will, however, facilitate the diagnosis and sometimes the definitive surgical treatment of selected cases by providing direct access to this complex joint with minimal associated morbidity.

REFERENCES

1. Takagi K. The arthroscope: the second report. Nippon Seikeigeka Gakkai Zasshi 1939B;14:441.
2. Watanabe M. Arthroscopy of small joints. Tokyo: Igakui-Shoin, 1985:7.
3. Whipple TL, Marotta J, Powell J. Techniques of wrist arthroscopy. Arthroscopy 1986;2(4):244.

BIBLIOGRAPHY

Chen YC. Arthroscopy of the wrist and finger joints. Orthop Clin North Am 1979;10(3):723.

2

Preoperative Evaluation and Imaging

*T*he wrist is a complex and compact region of anatomy and can be a difficult joint to evaluate clinically. Accurate diagnosis requires differentiation of intraarticular symptoms from extraarticular symptoms and discrimination between symptomatic pathology and irrelevant incidental findings. Modern imaging techniques can be expensive as well as inconvenient. Clinicians should ensure that a patient's symptoms justify the cost of pursuing an elusive diagnosis.

Table 2-1 lists the available options for evaluating wrist problems. The use of these special procedures in the evaluation of wrist disorders depends on the examiner's clinical impressions. The list of differential diagnoses may dictate the use of these modalities in one order or another. Associated expense and risk of these procedures, as well as the degree of urgency for establishing a conclusive diagnosis, should also be taken into consideration in the selection of appropriate tests. The order of diagnostic procedures, therefore, will vary depending on the circumstances of each individual case and on the clinician's evaluation of cost and risk compared to potential benefit. It is important to understand the limitations as well as the potential of these diagnostic procedures, and to use them in ways that will result in the most expedient and cost-effective diagnosis rather than attempting to follow a rigid diagnostic algorithm. Any number of diagnostic pathways may be appropriate. In this regard, there is no other substitute for good clinical judgment.

HISTORY

Patients typically present with symptoms that relate to one or more of the following categories: pain, swelling, limitation of motion, deformity, pseudolocking, nonpainful clicking, or crepitus. It is important to ascertain whether pain is constant or intermittent, and whether it is aggravated or relieved by any specific position or activity.

Loss of motion in one or more planes should be distinguished as active or passive restriction. One should also determine whether the motion is

Table 2–1.

DIAGNOSTIC OPTIONS FOR THE EVALUATION
OF WRIST SYMPTOMS

- History
- Physical examination
- Static radiographs
- Motion series radiographs
- Selective injections
- Examination under Bier block anesthesia
- Fluoroscopic examination
- Arthrography
- Tomography
- Technetium-99 bone scan
- Gallium bone scan
- Computerized tomography
- Magnetic resonance imaging
- Arthroscopy
- Exploratory surgery

restricted by pain or by mechanical blocking. Similarly, swelling may be constant or intermittent. It may also be localized or generalized, and it is important to know whether or not it is activity related.

Deformity may be congenital, insidious, or traumatic in onset. A patient's interpretation of deformity and its onset must be known to the physician. I am reminded of a patient with bilateral asymptomatic Madelung's deformity who presented with concern about a large dorsal ganglion that caused her wrist to look abnormal.

Pseudolocking refers to a temporary acute loss of motion in all planes. It may be caused by carpal instability or by some other tissue interposition in the joint. When muscles are relaxed, the episode passes. However, in the event of intraarticular fracture or carpal dislocation, true locking may occur when wrist motion is mechanically blocked—even under anesthesia. Sounds emanating from the wrist are frequent, disconcerting symptoms, and any scraping or friction sounds merit investigation. Nonpainful clicking, however, can be ignored. It is not uncommon for the extensor carpi ulnaris (ECU) tendon to click on pronation and supination of the forearm. Clicking may also result from articular defects, carpal instability, and tears in the triangular fibrocartilage (TFC) complex. However, if sensibility is normal and there is no associated pain, these causes of wrist clicking can almost always be safely treated by reassuring the patient.

While obtaining the patient's history related to specific symptoms, ascertain the duration of symptoms and any events related to the onset. In cases of accident or trauma, recreate the mechanism of injury as accurately as possible. For symptoms of insidious onset, be sure to take a careful family history for similar symptoms or generalized joint disease, a work history, a history of prior injury such as fracture, and a general review of systems or symptoms in other joints that might indicate systemic disorders.

Patients are often able to localize their symptoms in the wrist and should be encouraged to do so as specifically as possible. Once focused on a particular anatomic region, the examiner can evaluate each potentially offending structure (Table 2-2). This concept of regional assessment of the wrist is especially rewarding. The anatomy of the wrist is complex, and even the simplest motion and loading patterns entail integrated carpal movements or compression. Generalized evaluation of pain, swelling, friction, movement, restriction, deformity, or strength will therefore provide only superficial information about wrist disorders.

PHYSICAL EXAMINATION

To identify specific abnormalities that require treatment, the examiner should be familiar with the integrated structures in the symptomatic anatomic region and examine each regional structure in turn. Associated regions should also be examined, but deliberate inventory of regional structures is most likely to lead to an accurate identification of suspected pathology and to differentiate between intraarticular and extraarticular pathology.

Unlike patients with abdominal, spinal, hip, or shoulder symptoms, patients with wrist problems are usually able to localize precisely the specific site of injury or pathology. The wrist is not disposed to radicular symptoms, referred pain, or to a vague distribution of pain within the joint, such as that which may be present in the hip or knee.

An exhaustive wrist examination is a tedious but usually rewarding exercise. With practice, it should be possible to develop a short and reasonably accurate list of differential diagnoses following a thorough examination. After the exam, the clinician should

Table 2–2.

WRIST STRUCTURES TO BE EVALUATED ACCORDING TO ANATOMIC REGION

Radial

Cutaneous neuromata
De Quervain's stenosing tenosynovitis
Other types of tenosynovitis
Radioscaphoid arthrosis involving styloid articulation
Scaphotrapeziotrapezoid (STT) arthrosis
Scaphoid fracture

Dorsal Radial

Cutaneous neuromata
Ganglion: intraarticular or extraarticular
Incipient ganglion
Bossing of metacarpal base
Extensor carpi radialis longus or brevis strain
  or rupture
Proximal scaphoid articular defect
Scapholunate ligament tear
Dynamic or static scapholunate dissociation
Fracture of radial styloid
Fracture of proximal pole of scaphoid

Dorsal

Extensor tenosynovitis
Capsule avulsion from lunate
Capsule avulsion from distal row
Lunate articular defect
Capitate articular defect
Lunocapitate arthrosis or scapholunate advanced
  collapsed wrist
Wrist synovitis (rheumatoid, other inflammatory)
Kienböck's disease
Fracture of distal radius
Fracture of lunate
Fracture of capitate

Dorsal Ulnar

Cutaneous neuromata
Subluxation of extensor carpi ulnaris
Retinaculum tear of extensor carpi ulnaris
Extensor carpi ulnaris tenosynovitis
Ruptured extensor junctura
Distal radioulnar joint dissociation
Distal radioulnar joint loose body
Distal radioulnar joint arthrosis
Torn triangular fibrocartilage complex
Lunotriquetral dissociation or ligament tear
Midcarpal instability
Articular defect, proximal pole of hamate
Fracture of ulnar styloid
Fracture of triquetrum
Fracture of hamate
Ulnocarpal impaction or abutment syndrome

Volar Ulnar

Pisotriquetral ligament tear
Fracture of pisiform
Flexor carpi ulnaris tendonitis or strain
Ulnar artery thrombosis; aneurysm
Ganglion
Ulnar tunnel compression
Articular defect, head of ulna
Ulnocarpal ligament tear

Volar

Fracture of hook of hamate
Ulnar neuromata
Flexor tenosynovitis
Flexor tendon strain or rupture
Rupture of palmaris longus
Lunate dislocation
Rupture of triquetro-hamate-capitate ligament
Carpal tunnel syndrome
Palmar cutaneous neuroma

Volar Radial

Ganglion
Radial artery thrombosis, aneurysm
Carpal tunnel syndrome
Rupture or sprain of volar radiocarpal ligament
Fracture of tubercle of trapezoid
Fracture of tubercle of scaphoid

consider using ancillary procedures when specifically indicated but not as a matter of routine or algorithmic compulsion.

Regional Examination

The patient should be seated for wrist examination with the elbow at the side and flexed 90° and with the palms open flat (Fig. 2-1). After surveying the hand and wrist for any evidence of swelling or change in contour, color, or temperature compared to the opposite wrist, the range of motion is measured. Compare pronation and supination. In neutral rotation, compare extension, flexion, and radial and ulnar deviation. Neutral forearm rotation and open palms allow easy reference for comparison of motion and measurement.

Dorsal Evaluation

Palpate all anatomic structures in an attempt to localize maximal tenderness. It is helpful to palpate each extensor tendon compartment respectfully, especially compartments one and six. Check for resistance to wrist extension when evaluating the extensor carpi radialis longus (ECRL) and extensor carpi radialis brevis (ECRB). Check for resistance to metaphalangeal (MP) joint extension when evaluating the extensor digitorum communis (EDC). The patient should hold the hand in an intrinsic

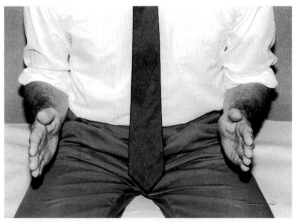

FIGURE 2–1.
Proper position for initial comparative range of motion assessment of the wrist. The patient is seated with palms open and forearms in neutral rotation.

minus position while the examiner attempts to depress each of the proximal phalanges.

Look for bossing at the base of the second and third metacarpals where the ECRL and ECRB attach. Palpate each articular margin and surface, including Lister's tubercle, the margins of the distal radius, and the proximal pole of the scaphoid and lunate. Examination of the scaphoid and lunate surfaces is facilitated by flexing the wrist. The proximal surfaces disappear in wrist extension (Fig. 2-2). Palpate the scapholunate interval between the third and fourth extensor compartments by positioning the wrist in slight flexion (Fig. 2-3). Flex the wrist acutely, and palpate the scapholunate ligament. With slight wrist flexion, palpate the lunotriquetral interval in line with the fourth ray. Certain carpal instabilities may cause pain localized to the dorsum of the wrist but will usually favor either the radial or ulnar side. Carpal instabilities will be discussed in Chapter 9.

The articular surface of the distal pole of the scaphoid can be palpated if the patient's thumb is opposed to the little finger with the wrist deviated in an ulnar direction (Fig. 2-4). The scaphotrapeziotrapezoid (STT) joint is a frequent site of degenerative arthrosis. Look for dorsal ganglia, usually found over the scapholunate interval between the third and fourth extensor compartments. Dorsal ganglia are accentuated clinically by flexion of the wrist (Fig. 2-5). Ganglia also can occasionally be found between the lunate and triquetrum in line with the fourth ray. A large dorsal ganglion may present two separate points of maximal tenderness if it arises beneath the common extensor retinaculum and presents proximally as well as distally at the edges of the retinaculum (*i.e.,* a "dumbbell" lesion; Fig. 2-6).

Radial Evaluation

Palpation for maximal tenderness is still the most revealing means of examining the wrist when symptoms are predominantly on the radial side. A radial examination should include the following:

Palpate the first extensor compartment, especially over the radial styloid.
Use Finkelstein's test. This procedure is less provocative if the patient is asked to do the test himself by grasping his thumb in his

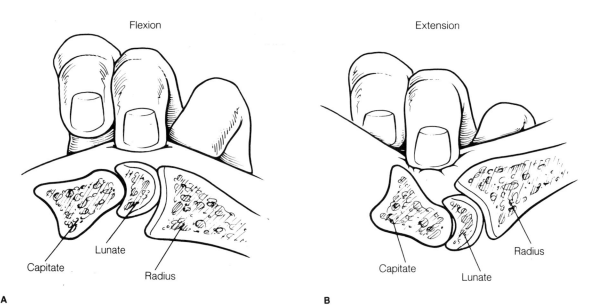

FIGURE 2–2.
Clinical assessment of lunate and scaphoid articular surfaces by palpation. (**A**) Flexion presents the articular surfaces dorsally.
(**B**) In extension, they are inaccessible.

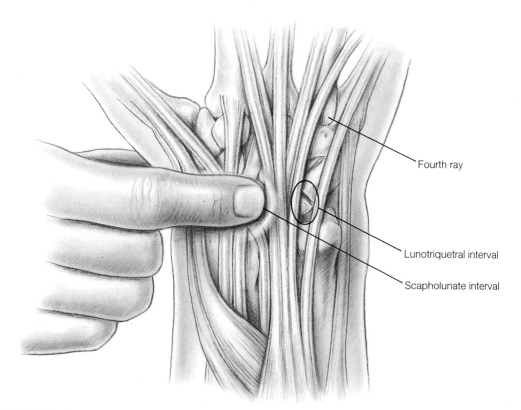

FIGURE 2–3.
With the wrist in slight flexion, the scapholunate interval can be palpated for tenderness between the third and fourth extensor compartments just distal to Lister's tubercle. With the wrist in flexion, the lunotriquetral interval can be palpated between the fourth and fifth extensor compartments in line with the fourth ray.

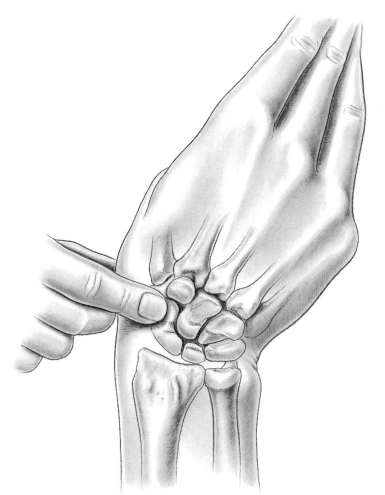

FIGURE 2–4.
Palpation of the distal pole of scaphoid for tenderness indicative of scaphotrapeziotrapezoid arthrosis. Thumb is opposed to little finger with wrist in ulnar deviation to present scaphoid articular surface dorsally.

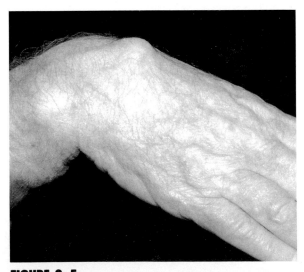

FIGURE 2–5.
Typical dorsal wrist ganglion accentuated by wrist flexion.

palm and simulating a hammering motion (Fig. 2-7).

Lightly palpate further proximally over the extensor pollicis brevis (EPB) and abductor pollicis longus (APL) while the thumb is actively moved to appreciate any bursal friction under the outcropping muscles (the so-called intersection syndrome sign; Fig. 2-8).

Examine the radial styloid for elongation or tenderness when palpated.

Look for radioscaphoid arthrosis, which is common with longstanding scapholunate dissociation. This is best evidenced clinically by tenderness over the radial styloid and may be accentuated by radial deviation of the wrist.

Scapholunate dissociation, as previously noted, may cause tenderness when dorsal palpation of the

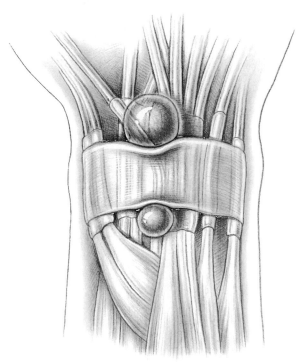

FIGURE 2–6.
Diagram of large dorsal ganglion arising beneath the common extensor retinaculum. It may present as a dumbbell lesion at the proximal and distal margins of retinaculum.

scapholunate interval is performed, especially if the wrist is in flexion. More subtle injury to the scapholunate ligament without complete dissociation of the scapholunate interval can be revealed by stressing the ligament. Watson described a provocative test for dynamic, or functional, scapholunate instability in which the scaphoid is held in a vertical position by applying pressure on the volar scaphoid tubercle.[1] As the wrist undergoes passive radial deviation (Fig. 2-9*A*), pain or slipping may be noted. I find that passive wrist flexion is as effective as radial deviation for this test, causing pain and forcing the proximal pole of the scaphoid to slip dorsally if instability is present (Fig. 2-9*B*).

Although grinding the first metacarpal against the trapezium has long been recommended as a means of assessing carpometacarpal (CMC) arthrosis, I have found it more reliable clinically to palpate the volar margin of the joint over the volar CMC ligament (Fig. 2-10). Tenderness in this area correlates well with CMC degenerative changes and is frequently present when the "grind" test is negative.

Localized tenderness on the radial side that does

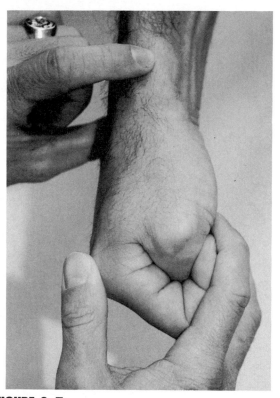

FIGURE 2–7.
Finkelstein's test. With the patient's thumb in palm, passive or active ulnar deviation elicits pain or tenderness where the first extensor compartment crosses the radial styloid.

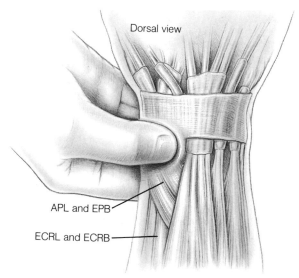

Dorsal view

APL and EPB

ECRL and ECRB

FIGURE 2–8.
Intersection syndrome. Palpation over the abductor pollicis longus (APL) and extensor pollicis brevis (EPB) as they cross the extensor carpi radialis longus (ECRL) and extensor carpi radialis brevis (ECRB) produces pain. Active thumb motion elicits a sensation of friction at this intersection.

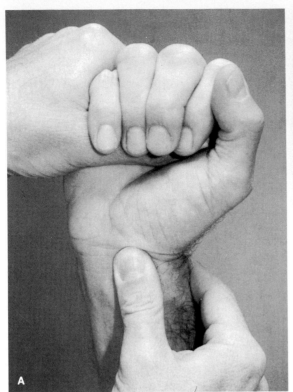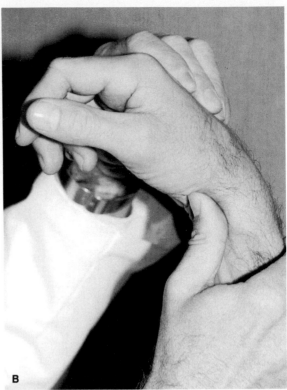

FIGURE 2–9.
Watson test for scapholunate instability. Examiner's thumb prevents distal pole of scaphoid from flexing as the wrist is (**A**) passively deviated radially or (**B**) passively flexed.

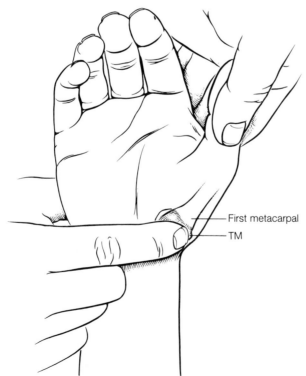

First metacarpal

TM

FIGURE 2–10.
Carpometacarpal (CMC) arthritis of the thumb most consistently causes tenderness to palpation over the volar CMC ligament. The thumb CMC joint is passively extended while the volar margin of the base of the first ray is palpated. (TM, trapezium.)

not occur directly over a tendon, ligament, or joint margin should raise the suspicion of a cutaneous neuroma. Percussion may cause a positive Tinel's sign. Usually there is some history of sharp or blunt trauma, such as a car hood or washing machine lid falling on the radial aspect of the wrist.

Ulnar Evaluation

There are many causes of ulnar wrist pain that are not easy to differentiate. For the ulnar area more than any other, position is most relevant in evaluating pain.

Extensor carpi ulnaris tendinitis or subluxation is very common. The ECU tendon frequently snaps audibly with supination. Unless it is painful, the snapping is of no concern. Remember that the ECU is in its shortest configuration and takes its most direct course with the forearm in pronation. It is stressed through its most tortuous course in supination (Fig. 2-11). It is further stressed during flexion and radial deviation with supination. If ulnar

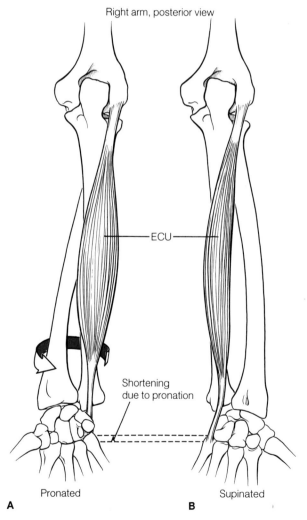

Right arm, posterior view

ECU

Shortening due to pronation

A Pronated   B Supinated

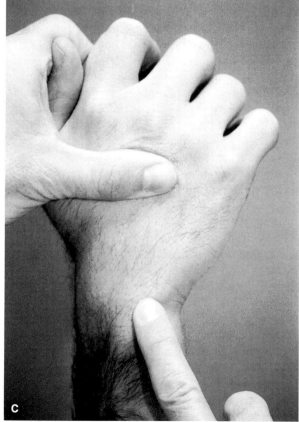

C

FIGURE 2–11.

Diagram representing the effect of pronation and supination on the extensor carpi ulnaris (ECU). (**A**) In pronation, the radiocarpal level is closer to the elbow, and the ECU is shorter and takes a straighter, more relaxed course from origin to insertion. (**B**) In supination, the radiocarpal distance to the elbow is lengthened, and the ECU is stretched and takes an oblique course from the lateral elbow epicondyle to the medial side of the hand. (**C**) For clinical examination of the ECU, place the tendon under strain by elbow extension, forearm supination, and wrist flexion. Then palpate the ECU within its retinaculum at the head of the ulna.

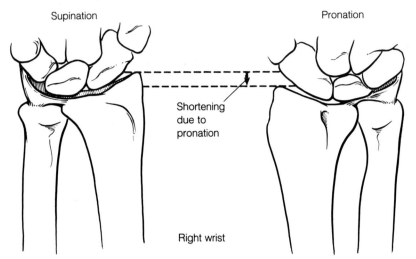

Supination

Pronation

Shortening
due to
pronation

Right wrist

FIGURE 2–12.
Ulnocarpal abutment is accentuated by pronation, which places the radius in an oblique position relative to the ulna. This shortens the elbow–carpal distance relative to the length of the ulna and compresses the triangular fibrocartilage articular disc between the ulna and lunate. Ulnocarpal abutment is further accentuated by radial deviation of the wrist.

wrist pain in these positions is aggravated by palpation of the sixth extensor compartment, ECU tendinitis or subluxation should be suspected.

Lesions of the triangular fibrocartilage complex (TFCC) are the next most common cause of ulnar wrist symptoms. Tears should be suspected if tenderness is present between the head of the ulna and triquetrum. This area should be palpated in pronation and in supination. Remember that pronation shortens the radius relative to the ulna and increases compression of the TFC articular disc between the ulna and triquetrum (Fig. 2-12). This area should also be gently palpated as the wrist is repeatedly deviated toward the ulna to appreciate subtle stutters or clicks in the motion.

Ligamentous portions of the TFCC are subject to injury with violent wrist extension or radial deviation. This usually involves the volar ulnocarpal ligaments (Fig. 2-13), which will be tender when palpated over the volar aspect of the ulnocarpal interval in supination and extension. While the TFCC does participate in pronation and supination of the wrist, it is hazardous to ascribe pronation and supination pain to lesions of the TFC.

There are three patterns of carpal instability that can cause pain on the ulnar side of the wrist: pisotriquetral instability, lunotriquetral instability, and midcarpal instability (MCI). Pisotriquetral ligament injuries are evidenced by pain or by displacement of the pisiform. Less severe injuries to the pisohamate ligament or to the pisotriquetral joint capsule should

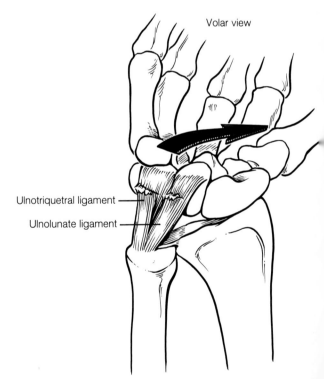

Volar view

Ulnotriquetral ligament

Ulnolunate ligament

FIGURE 2–13.
Mechanism of injury to the volar ulnocarpal ligaments. Ulnotriquetral ligaments and ulnolunate ligaments are occasionally avulsed from the ulna in association with injuries to the distal radioulnar joint, but are more commonly torn at the level of the proximal carpal row by forceful extension and radial deviation of the wrist.

be suspected if resistance to flexion and ulnar deviation of the wrist through the flexor carpi ulnaris tendon causes pain.

Lunotriquetral instability is due to disruption of the interosseous lunotriquetral ligament and may cause tenderness over this interval when dorsal palpation is performed. The Shuck test, a provocative maneuver that translates the lunate and triquetrum in opposite directions in the sagittal plane, may further isolate the offending joint (Fig. 2-14). It is easy to feel the ulnar surface of the triquetrum. Pressing this surface in a radial direction will also accentuate the pain of lunotriquetral instability (Fig. 2-15).

Midcarpal instability occurs when the strong volar ligament between the triquetrum, hamate, and capitate is ruptured or stretched (Fig. 2-16). Midcarpal instability may be an extension of lunotri-

quetral instability, as the two are frequently seen in association. The volar triquetro-hamate-capitate (THC) ligament is protected by the hook of the hamate, however, and is not palpable. Clinical demonstration of MCI requires coaching the patient to clench the fist tightly and then to deviate the fist toward the ulnar as in hammering or swinging a bat or golf club with the leading hand (Fig. 2-17). With MCI there is a palpable and visible clunk or shift of

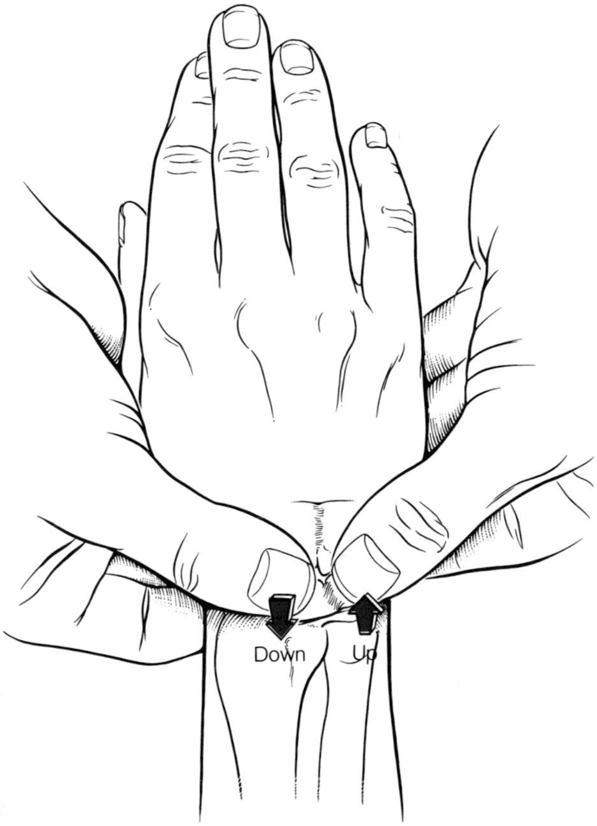

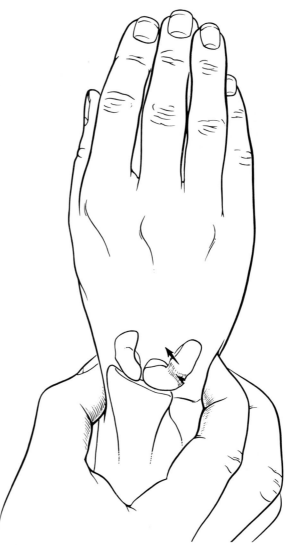

FIGURE 2–14.
The Shuck test. The pisiform and triquetrum are passively translated dorsally and toward the volar relative to the lunate. Positioning the wrist in slight flexion improves the examiner's grip on the lunate.

FIGURE 2–15.
The squeeze test for lunotriquetral (LT) instability. Note the oblique orientation of the LT articulation. Squeezing the proximal row in the coronal plane with the examiner's finger on the ulnar side of the triquetrum shifts the triquetrum distally, reproducing pain if the LT interval is unstable.

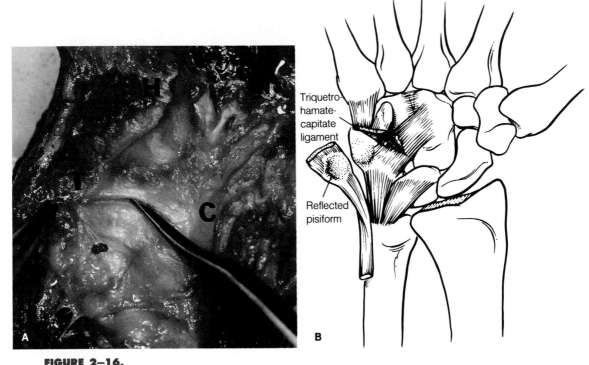

FIGURE 2—16.
Volar triquetro-hamate-capitate (THC) ligament (right wrist). This bold, distinct ligament regulates midcarpal stability. (**A**) Dissected specimen. Note hook of hamate (H), triquetral insertion (T), and capitate insertion (C). (**B**) Diagrammatic representation of THC ligament rupture. This can sometimes be seen arthroscopically in the midcarpal space.

the carpus in which the ulnar side of the carpus appears to drop toward the palm.

This shift represents several intercarpal events. With loss of the ligament constraint between the triquetrum and hamate, ulnar deviation allows the

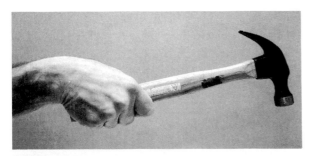

FIGURE 2—17.
Midcarpal instability demonstrated clinically by the swing of a hammer. Symptoms are aggravated by power grip with ulnar deviation. Similar motions are reproduced by the leading hand in the swing of a bat or golf club. Volar shift of the ulnar side of the carpus can be observed clinically.

proximal pole of the hamate to slide dorsally and radially on the saddle of the triquetrum. The proximal pole of the hamate "hangs" on the ulnar edge of the lunate when the fist is clenched. The sudden shift occurring with ulnar deviation represents the lunate moving suddenly into a dorsal intercalated segmental instability (DISI) orientation (Fig. 2-18). The proximal pole of the hamate and capitate shift dorsally as the distal row flexes, causing the ulnar side of the carpus to appear to drop toward the palm (Fig. 2-19).

The distal radioulnar joint (DRUJ) is an interesting joint with a complex combination of pronation and supination as well as translational motion in the sagittal plane. Again, tenderness on palpation is an important observation. Explore the dorsal interval between the radius and ulna through a range of pronation and supination. Volar and dorsal translation excursion should be compared with the opposite wrist in neutral rotation. Prominence of the head of the ulna should also be compared with the

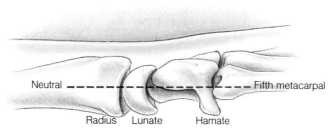

Ulnar view

Normal

Neutral - Fifth metacarpal

Radius   Lunate   Hamate

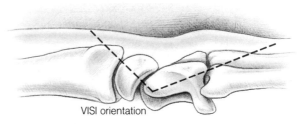

MCI in neutral deviation

VISI orientation

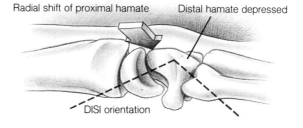

MCI in ulnar deviation

Radial shift of proximal hamate   Distal hamate depressed

DISI orientation

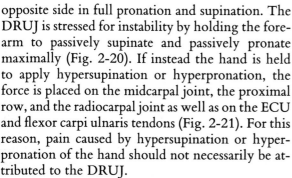

FIGURE 2–18.

Lunate pivot shift with midcarpal instability (MCI). Passively, the lunate assumes volar intercalated segmental instability (VISI) orientation, producing an extension posture between the proximal and distal rows. With compression and ulnar deviation, the proximal pole of hamate slides dorsally and radially with a subsequent shift of the lunate from VISI to dorsal intercalated segmental instability (DISI), with a flexion posture between proximal and distal rows.

opposite side in full pronation and supination. The DRUJ is stressed for instability by holding the forearm to passively supinate and passively pronate maximally (Fig. 2-20). If instead the hand is held to apply hypersupination or hyperpronation, the force is placed on the midcarpal joint, the proximal row, and the radiocarpal joint as well as on the ECU and flexor carpi ulnaris tendons (Fig. 2-21). For this reason, pain caused by hypersupination or hyperpronation of the hand should not necessarily be attributed to the DRUJ.

The DRUJ can be compressed by squeezing the ulnar head into the sigmoid notch of the radius. If the forearm is pronated and supinated with such

pressure applied, pain may be reproduced in the presence of DRUJ arthrosis.

Clinical evaluation of the ulnar side of the wrist also requires careful palpation and percussion of the cutaneous branches of the ulnar nerve.

Volar Evaluation

Volar wrist symptoms are not difficult to differentiate clinically. Flexor tendinitis or various degrees of rupture of the flexor tendons can be assessed by resisting the pull of each tendon respectively to reproduce pain.

Ulnar artery aneurysms are not uncommon.

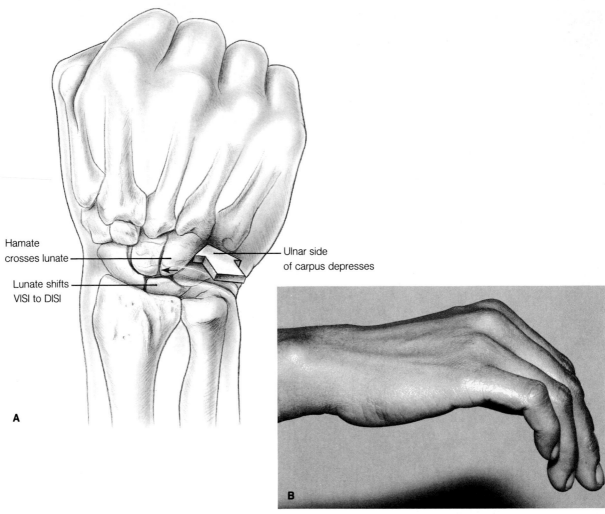

Hamate
crosses lunate

Lunate shifts
VISI to DISI

Ulnar side
of carpus depresses

A

B

FIGURE 2–19.
Midcarpal instability. (**A**) Clinical testing with power grip in ulnar deviation causes the ulnar side of the carpus to appear to drop toward the palm or to supinate. (**B**) Photograph of volar subluxation of the ulnar side of the carpus. (DISI, dorsal intercalated segmental instability; VISI, volar intercalated segmental instability.)

They present with pain and usually a pulsatile mass on the volar ulnar aspect of the wrist (Fig. 2-22). Similarly, radial artery aneurysms or arteriovenous (AV) malformations are usually tender when palpated, soft and bulky, and pulsatile. With a doppler examination, one can usually hear a bruit over arterial lesions at the wrist.

The differentiation of carpal tunnel syndrome from other wrist disorders should not be difficult. Pain or dysesthesias usually radiate distally in the pattern of distribution of the median nerve and proximally up the volar aspect of the forearm. Phalen's test (Fig. 2-23) or Tinel's sign may be positive, and the two-point discrimination test in the median nerve distribution may be increased. The examiner should also check for evidence of thenar atrophy (Fig. 2-24). Volar radiocarpal ligament injuries may be difficult to assess clinically. Reproduction of pain during wrist extension, especially with radial deviation, will be helpful, particularly if there is ten-

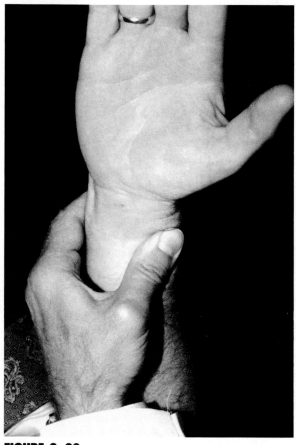

FIGURE 2–20.

The distal radioulnar joint is stressed clinically by passive supination applied through the forearm.

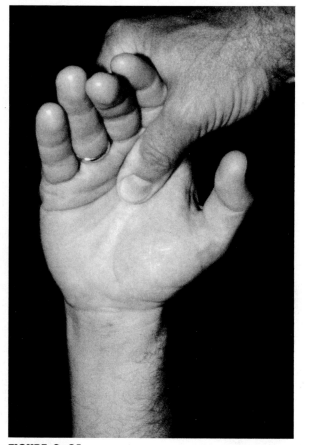

FIGURE 2–21.

Radiocarpal instability is stressed clinically by hypersupination applied through the hand.

derness when palpation is performed over the volar aspect of the radial styloid where these ligaments arise (Fig. 2-25).

Radiographs

Routine radiographic views of the wrist should include a posteroanterior (PA) projection with the forearm in neutral rotation, a lateral projection with the forearm in neutral rotation, and a scaphoid oblique projection with the forearm in 30° to 40° of supination (Fig. 2-26). When carpal instability or ulnocarpal abutment is suspected, a motion series is helpful. The motion series should include flexion and extension lateral projections and PA projections

in radial and ulnar deviation with a clenched fist to accentuate carpal dissociation patterns (Fig. 2-27). Finally, carpal tunnel view will allow visualization of the hook of the hamate and the volar lip of the radius (Fig. 2-28).

Selective Injections

Selectively anesthetizing specific tissues of the wrist will help to differentiate between intraarticular and extraarticular symptom sources. It may be difficult to differentiate, for example, between tendinitis of the ECU and some intraarticular inflammatory synovitis on the ulnar side. Injection of 1% lidocaine

(text continues on page 28)

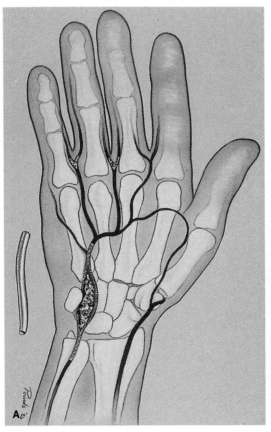

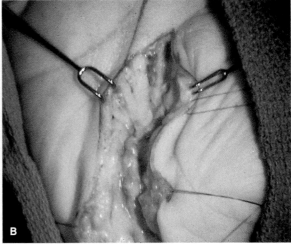

FIGURE 2–22.
Ulnar artery aneurysm. (**A**) Typical location of aneurysm (right wrist). (**B**) Photograph of aneurysm in same location. (Courtesy of L. Andrew Koman, M.D., Bowman Gray School of Medicine, Winston-Salem, NC.)

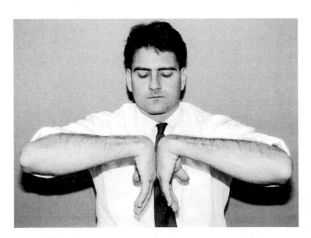

FIGURE 2–23.
Phalen's test for carpal tunnel syndrome. Acute flexion presses the median nerve beneath the transverse carpal ligament.

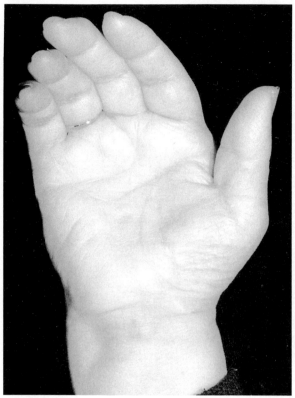

FIGURE 2–24.
Thenar atrophy secondary to carpal tunnel syndrome.

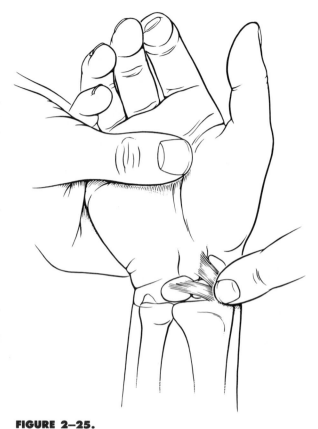

FIGURE 2–25.
Sprains of the volar radiocarpal ligaments. The examiner holds the wrist in extension and palpates the origin of the ligaments on the volar aspect of the radial styloid. Passive ulnar deviation aggravates injuries to the radioscaphocapitate. Passive radial deviation aggravates injuries to the radiolunotriquetral ligament.

FIGURE 2–26.
Standard radiograph series of the wrist includes posteroanterior (PA) in neutral forearm rotation and neutral wrist position, lateral projection with metacarpals parallel to axis of the radius, and scaphoid view taken in PA projection with forearm supinated 30° to 40° and wrist in ulnar deviation (typical handwriting position).

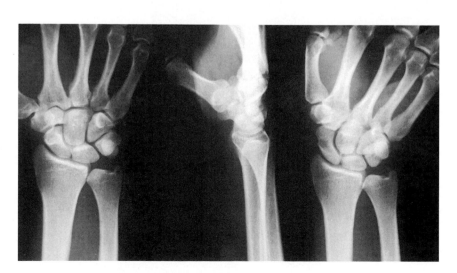

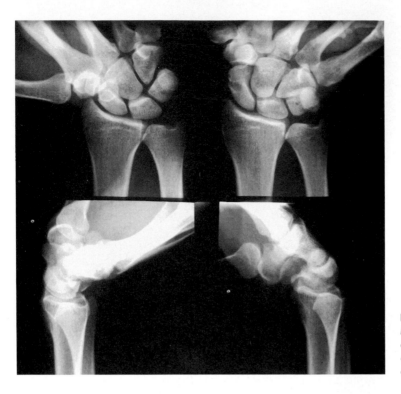

FIGURE 2–27.
Motion series in full radial and full ulnar deviation, and laterally in full extension and flexion. Note change in position of scaphoid with radial and ulnar deviation.

(Xylocaine) into the ECU tendon sheath will temporarily relieve any tendon discomfort without affecting potential intraarticular lesions. Bone pain and pain caused by articular defects are not reliably alleviated by intraarticular injections; however, pain

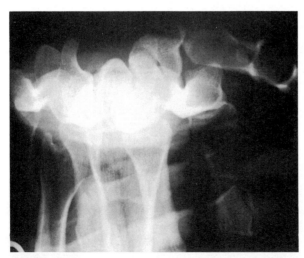

FIGURE 2–28.
Carpal tunnel view demonstrates hook of hamate and smooth contour of carpal canal.

caused by loose bodies, inflammatory synovitis, and mechanical defects in the joint is relieved by these injections.

Differential nerve blocks can assist the clinician as well. They are especially useful in identifying malingering patients or those with psychosomatic syndromes. One must be adept at selectively blocking the median nerve, the ulnar nerve, and the radial cutaneous branches to use this technique with confidence. If complete motor block of the median nerve is achieved but the patient still perceives pain in the median nerve distribution, continued pursuit of an anatomic cause of these symptoms is likely to be futile unless brachial plexus or cervical root pathology are present.

Examination Under Bier Block

Intravenous Bier block anesthesia can be used safely in a clinical setting to facilitate physical examination for mechanical wrist problems. When it is difficult to differentiate between loss of motion secondary to pain, pseudolocking, and contracture, administration of Bier block will provide complete sensory and motor anesthesia for an uninhibited examination of the wrist. Restricted motion under Bier block will be the result of joint contracture or mechanical derangement. The block also provides an opportunity for manipulation of the wrist under anesthesia.

I have found this technique to be especially useful in the evaluation of postoperative patients who are progressing slowly and in the examination of patients with suspected hysterical conversion. One should be familiar with the technique and risks of administering intravenous blocks and should have available the appropriate drugs and equipment in the event of cardiac arrhythmia or seizure.

Examination Under Fluoroscopy

Small fluoroscopic units suitable for office use are extremely useful for evaluating the wrist in certain circumstances. Fluoroscopic examination is valuable in the evaluation of cases of MCI or other carpal dissociation patterns when plain film motion series are insufficient to establish a diagnosis. Fluoroscopy is also useful to help localize the presence of loose or foreign bodies in the wrist. This means of examination is far less expensive than cineradiography, and the test can be performed and the results interpreted by the clinician.

ARTHROGRAPHY

Defects of the articular disc of the TFCC and most tears in the intrinsic ligaments of the wrist will be revealed by arthrography. Double contrast studies are not recommended for the wrist because foaming or bubble formation will interfere with interpretation of the films. Only a small volume of contrast medium is required; usually 1 to 1.5 ml is sufficient. Larger volumes can cause painful extravasation into subcutaneous tissues and may mask subtle evidence of intraarticular pathology (Fig. 2-29).

Radiocarpal space injections are used primarily to detect defects in the TFC. X-ray films should include oblique projections to identify capsular diverticuli other than the prestyloid recess, especially on the ulnar side of the wrist. Midcarpal space injection is the best method for identifying tears in the scapholunate or lunotriquetral ligaments,

whereas the radiocarpal space injection will show most of the ligament lesions. A valve effect may be present, and the dye from a radiocarpal space injection will not pass through the tear as readily as it does with midcarpal space injections (Fig. 2-30). Injection of contrast solutions into the DRUJ will help to identify loose bodies in that space. This injection is also useful for detecting the presence of TFCC tears if the radiocarpal space injection is negative (Fig. 2-29C). It is not necessary to routinely perform three-compartment arthrography. Injection of specific compartments should be requested by the examiner based on clinical diagnostic impressions.

Roth has reported a controlled study in which arthroscopy proved to be more sensitive than arthrography for identifying tears of the TFCC.[2] Nevertheless, I find arthrography valuable before arthroscopy when the clinical diagnostic impression is questionable or incomplete and in situations where the arthroscopic examination is expected to be difficult, as in the case of very petite wrists or patients who have had previous surgical arthrotomy. In such circumstances, it is helpful to have as much preoperative diagnostic information as possible.

TOMOGRAPHY

Since the advent of computed tomography (CT) scans, plain tomograms are of little benefit except in the assessment of fracture healing or the healing progress of intercarpal fusions. In these cases, trispiral tomography is an accurate and less expensive means of evaluating new bone formation.

COMPUTED TOMOGRAPHY

Computed tomography of the wrist can be obtained in three planes. The primary advantage of CT over trispiral tomography is the ability to provide transverse cuts of the wrist. Although soft tissues can be seen with CT scans, resolution is rarely adequate for soft-tissue diagnosis, except to confirm the presence of large cysts or soft masses. The procedure, however, is especially effective for certain skeletal disorders. Small occult fractures of the carpal bones can be identified using 1-mm serial cuts. Intraartic-

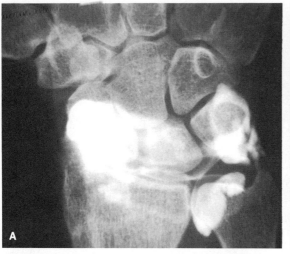
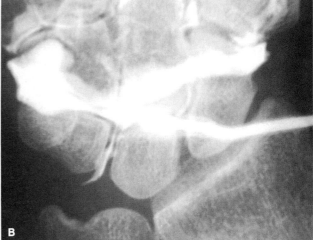
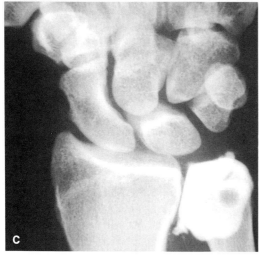

FIGURE 2–29.

Three-phase arthrogram. (**A**) Radiocarpal injection demonstrates defect in triangular fibrocartilage complex. (**B**) Midcarpal space injection demonstrates intact lunotriquetral ligament. (**C**) Distal radioulnar joint (DRUJ) injection confirms the integrity of the triangular fibrocartilage complex if radiocarpal injection is negative. May also demonstrate void in the dye representing loose bodies in DRUJ.

ular fractures of the distal radius are evaluated best by this technique to assess the extent of combination and displacement of articular fragments (Fig. 2-31). In cases of suspected DRUJ subluxation, CT scans obtained in pronation and supination will show clearly the ulna in relation to the sigmoid notch of the radius.

One should always obtain comparative views of the opposite extremity. For optimal studies, the technician or radiologist should ensure that the forearms are parallel to each other in the gantry so perfectly transverse cuts are obtained (Fig. 2-32). The alignment of the right and left wrists should be as similar as possible for comparison of the same levels on each side.

CINERADIOGRAPHY

Dynamic instabilities of the wrist can be extremely difficult to diagnose. When there is no fixed deformity or malalignment between carpals, plain radiographs will appear normal. Motion series of extreme positions may show only subtle or equivocal abnormalities. Injuries to the scapholunate or lunotriquetral intrinsic ligaments and volar THC extrinsic ligament, among others, can cause symptomatic shifts between carpal bones that occur suddenly during the course of certain wrist motions. These shifts cannot be appreciated with still-frame imaging, but may be evident with fluoroscopic examination as noted above (Fig. 2-33). For docu-

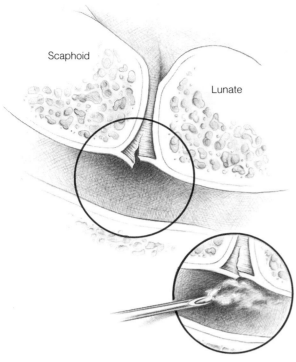

Scaphoid

Lunate

FIGURE 2–30.

Diagram of the valve effect that may cause negative arthrogram with radiocarpal space injection when scapholunate or lunotriquetral ligaments are torn. Positive pressure in the radiocarpal space closes the defect. A subsequent midcarpal space injection is recommended.

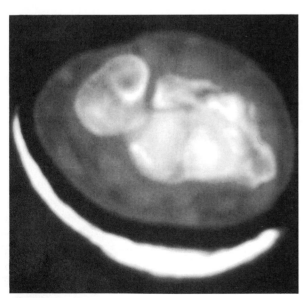

FIGURE 2–31.

This computed tomography scan of an articular fracture of the right distal radius (pronation) demonstrates the number, size, and degree of displacement of articular fragments preoperatively.

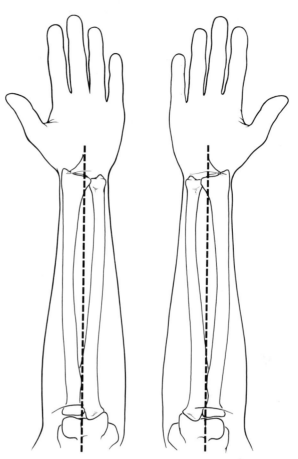

FIGURE 2–32.

The proper position of forearms in the computed tomography gantry. Elbows should be together with forearms parallel in supination, neutral position, or pronation. A common technical error is to position the patient with arms overhead, elbows at shoulder width, and wrists together. This improper positioning will produce oblique cuts through the distal radioulnar joint.

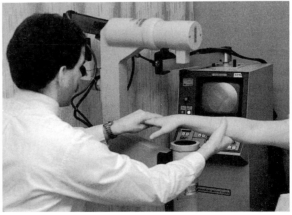

FIGURE 2–33.

Fluoroscopic examination of the wrist. Low radiation output and virtually no scatter minimizes exposure and provides high resolution motion studies of the carpus (Courtesy of HealthMate, Northbrook, IL).

mentation, more intensive study, and to reduce radiation exposure, fluoroscopic examinations captured on videotape or film are extremely useful.

The availability of videotape technology has made this diagnostic modality much more convenient than celluloid film, which requires projection. Compact, low-dose radiation fluoroscopic units are now available, which, when coupled with a videotape recorder, make cineradiography a convenient and reasonable office procedure.

TECHNETIUM-99 BONE SCAN

The use of technetium-99 radioisotope scans are invaluable in the evaluation of subtle or obscure disorders of the wrist. The isotope concentrates in areas of increased blood flow or inflammation (Fig. 2-34). This test provides an excellent screening mechanism for localization of pathologic change when vague or inconsistent symptoms preclude a focused evaluation. Pinhole views provide magnification of the image and should be requested in PA and lateral projections of both wrists for comparison.

GALLIUM SCANS

Isotopes of gallium seek white blood cells. Gallium scans are rarely necessary in the wrist, but this is a very sensitive means of detecting wrist infections, especially osteomyelitis.

MAGNETIC RESONANCE IMAGING

As in other anatomic regions, magnetic resonanace imaging (MRI) studies of the wrist are becoming increasingly helpful and common. Magnetic resonance imaging provides the most effective noninvasive means of evaluating soft-tissue lesions and circulation disorders of bone (Fig. 2-35).

The continuing development of more effective magnetic coils for the wrist is providing MRI images of higher resolution. The interpretation of MRI studies, however, requires unique expertise. The soft-tissue anatomy of the wrist is complex, and the relationship of these structures is not always familiar to those who perform or interpret the studies. Im-

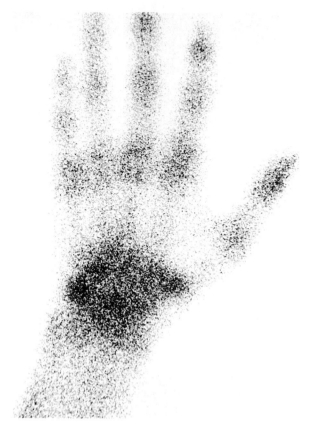

FIGURE 2–34.
Technetium-99 bone scan demonstrates diffuse increased isotope concentration throughout the carpus, with greatest focal concentration on the ulnar side over the triangular fibrocartilage complex.

ages should be enlarged enough to permit identification of the anatomic source of recorded signals when soft-tissue pathology is suspected. An MRI is an ideal means of reflecting bone density and viability. Osteonecrosis following scaphoid or capitate fractures or Kienböck's disease is most effectively identified on MRI by the contrasting signals produced on the T2-weighted images (Fig. 2-36).

ANGIOGRAPHY

Although angiography in the upper extremities is used primarily to evaluate circulatory disorders in the hand, it is especially useful on certain occasions in the wrist as well. It is the most effective means for diagnosing and evaluating the size and com-

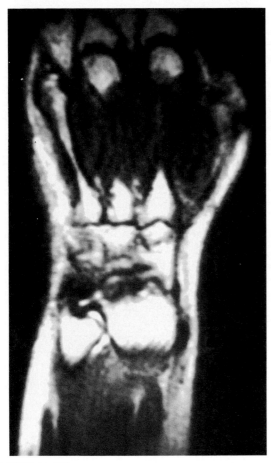

FIGURE 2–35.
A magnetic resonance imaging film delineating soft tissues of the wrist. Fluid density represents normal bone and fluid accumulation (effusion) adjacent to the triangular fibrocartilage complex.

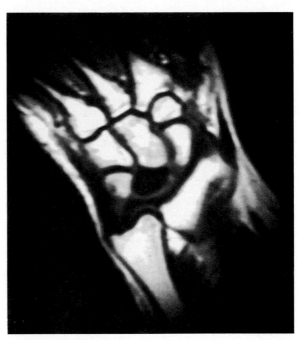

FIGURE 2–36.
A magnetic resonance imaging film of Kienböck's disease. Loss of fluid signal from lunate demonstrates loss of vascularity.

REFERENCES

1. Taleisnik J. The wrist. New York: Churchill-Livingstone, 1985:247.
2. Roth JH, Haddad RG. Radiocarpal arthroscopy and arthrography in the diagnosis of ulnar wrist pain. Arthroscopy 1986;2(4):234.

BIBLIOGRAPHY

Beckenbaugh RD. Accurate evaluation and management of the painful wrist following injury: an approach to carpal instability. Orthop Clin North Am 1984;15(2): 289.
Beresina SJ, Vannier MW, Logan SE, Weeks PM. Three dimensional wrist imaging: evaluation of functional and pathologic anatomy by computer. Clin Plast Surg 1986;13(3):389.
Biondetti PR, Vannier MW, Gilula LA, Knapp R. Wrist coronal and transaxial CT scanning. Radiology 1987; 163(1):149.
Bottke CA, Louis DS, Braunstein EM. Diagnosis and treatment of obscure ulnar-sided wrist pain. Orthopedics 1989;8:1075.

munications of arteriovenous malformations, arterial aneurysms, thrombosis of the ulnar artery, and hemangiomas. Doppler examination of the radial and ulnar arteries provides general impressions about blood flow, but definitive study of vascular lesions is accomplished best with angiography.

ULTRASONOGRAPHY

At present, ultrasonography has few applications in the examination of the wrist. Soft-tissue disorders are much better evaluated by MRI, even with its limitations.

Brown DE, Lichtman DM. The evaluation of chronic wrist pain. Orthop Clin North Am 1984;15(2):183.

Brumfield RH, Champoux JA. A biomechanical study of normal wrist motion. Clin Orthop 1984;187:23.

Bush CH, Gillespy T III, Dell PC. High resolution CT of the wrist: initial experience with scaphoid disorders and surgical fusions. AJR 1987;149(4):757.

Carlson JD, Trombley CA. The effect of wrist immobilization on performance of the Jebsen hand function test. Am J Occup Ther 1983;37(3):167.

Carroll RE, Coyle MP Jr. Dysfunction of the pisotriquetral joint: treatment by excision of the pisiform. J Hand Surg [Am] 1985;10(5):703.

Cone RO, Szabo R, Resnick D, Gelberman R, Talesnik J, Gilula LA. Computed tomography of the normal soft tissues of the wrist. Invest Radiol 1983;18(3):546.

Corley FG Jr. Examination and assessment of injuries and problems effecting the elbow, wrist and hand. Emerg Med Clin North Am 1984;2(2):295.

Czitrom AA, Lister GD. Measurement of grip strength in the diagnosis of wrist pain. J Hand Surg [Am] 1988;13(1):16.

DeLange A, Kauer JM, Huiskes R. Kinematic behavior of the human wrist joint: a roentgen-stereophotogrammetric analysis. J Orthop Res 1985;3(1):56.

Dell PC. Distal radioulnar joint dysfunction. Hand Clin 1987 3(4):563.

Eckhardt WA, Palmer AK. Recurrent dislocation of extensor carpi ulnaris tendon. J Hand Surg [Am] 1981; 6(6):629.

Fisk GR. An overview of injuries of the wrist. Clin Orthop 1980;149:137.

Fry HJ. Physical signs in the hand and wrist seen in the overuse injury syndrome of the upper limb. Aust NZ J Surg. 1986;56(1):47.

Garcia-Elias M, Dobyns JH, Cooney WP III, Linscheid RL. Traumatic axial dislocations of the carpus. J Hand Surg [Am] 1989;14(3):446.

Goodman ML, Shankman JB. Palmar dislocation of the trapezoid: a case report. J Hand Surg [Am] 1983;8(5): 606.

Green DP. The sore wrist without a fracture. Instr Course Lect 1985;34:300.

Hagert CJ. The distal radioulnar joint. Hand Clin 1987; 3(1):41.

Hamlin C. Diagnosis of wrist injuries. Emerg Med Clin North Am 1985;3(2):311.

Hankin FM, White SJ, Braunstein EM, Louis DS. Dynamic radiographic evaluation of obscure wrist pain in the teen-age patient. J Hand Surg [Am] 1987;11(6): 805.

Hoffman DS, Strick PL. Step-tracking movements of the wrist in humans: kinematic analysis. J Neurosci 1986; 6(11):3309.

Horger MM. The reliability of goniometric measurements of active and passive wrist motions. Am J Occup Ther 1990;44(4):342.

Kauer JM. Functional anatomy of the wrist. Clin Orthop 1988;149:9.

Kauer JM, DeLange A. The carpal joint: anatomy and function. Hand Clin 1987;3(1):23.

Kleinman WB. Management of chronic rotary subluxation of the scaphoid by scapho-trapezial-trapezoid arthrodesis: rationale for the technique, post-operative changes and biomechanics, and results. Hand Clin 1987;3(1):113.

Lakie M, Walsh EG, Wright GW. Passive mechanical properties of the wrist and physiological tremor. J Neurol Neurosurg Psychiatry 1986;49(6):669.

Linscheid RL, Dobyns JH. The unified concept of carpal injuries. Ann Chir Main 1984;3(1):35.

Mayfield JK. Mechanism of carpal injuries. Clin Orthop 1980;149:45.

Mayfield JK. Patterns of injuries to carpal ligaments: a spectrum. Clin Orthop 1984;187:36.

Merhar GL, Clark RA, Schneider HJ, Stern PJ. High resolution computed tomography in patients with a carpal tunnel syndrome. Skeletal Radiol 1986;15(7):549.

Nakamura R, Horii E, Tanaka Y, Imaeda T, Hayakawa N. Three dimensional CT imaging for wrist disorders. J Hand Surg [Br] 1989;14(1):53.

Nathan R, Lester B, Melone CP Jr. The acutely injured wrist: an anatomic basis for operative treatment. Orthop Rev 1987;16(6):401.

Neviaser RJ, Palmer AK. Traumatic perforation of the articular disk of the triangular fibrocartilage complex of the wrist. Bull Hosp Jt Dis Orthop Inst 1984;44(2): 376.

Paley D, McMurtry RY, Murray JF. Dorsal dislocation of the ulnar styloid and extensor carpi ulnaris tendon into the distal radioulnar joint: the empty sulcis sign. J Hand Surg [Am] 1986;12(6):1029.

Palmer AK. The distal radioulnar joint: anatomy, biomechanics, and triangular fibrocartilage complex abnormalities. Hand Clin 1987;3(1):31.

Palmer AK, Levinsohn EM, Kuzma GR. Arthrography of the wrist. J Hand Surg [Am] 1983;8(1):15.

Palmer AK, Werner FW, Murphy D, Glisson R. Functional wrist motion: a biomechanical study. J Hand Surg [Am] 1985;10(1):39.

Pasila M, Karaharju EO, Lepisto PV. Reliability of the physical test and examination of the wrist. Ann Chir Gynaecol 1973;62(6):334.

Ranawat CS, Harrison MO, Jordan LR. Arthrography of the wrist joint. Clin Orthop 1972;83:6.

Sadr B, Lalehzaria M. Traumatic avulsion of the tendon of extensor carpi radialis longus. J Hand Surg [Am] 1987;12(6):1035.

Tehranzadeh J, Labosky DA. Detection of intraarticular loose osteochondral fragments by double contrast wrist arthrography: a case report of a basketball injury. Am J Sports Med 1984;12(1):77.

Vance RM, Gelberman RH, Evans EF. Scaphocapitate fractures: patterns of dislocation, mechanisms of injury, and preliminary results of treatment. J Bone Joint Surg [Am] 1980;62(2):271.

Watson HK. Examination of the scaphoid. J Hand Surg [Am] 1988;13(5):657.

Watson HK, Black DM. Instabilities of the wrist. Hand Clin 1987;3(1):103–111.

Watson HK, Brenner LH. Degenerative disorders of the wrist. J Hand Surg [Am] 1985;10:102.

Weber ER. Concept governing the rotational shift of the intercalated segment of the carpus. Orthop Clin North Am 1984;15(2):193.

Zemel NP. Prevention and treatment of complications from fractures of the distal radius and ulna. Hand Clin 1987;3(1):1.

3

Instrumentation

*S*urgical arthroscopy of the wrist requires a number of specialized instruments. A few of these instruments represent mere size reductions of instruments used for knee or shoulder arthroscopy. Others embody specific design features to accommodate the consistency of tissues in the wrist or the necessary angles of surgical approach.

The space required to manipulate instruments within the wrist joint is obtained by placing traction on the fingers. Distending the joint with infusion of fluid or gas will not provide adequate space between the radius and carpus or between the proximal and distal carpal rows, even under reasonable pressure. In most cases, traction equal to or 1 to 2 pounds more than the weight of the arm will provide enough space between articular surfaces to manipulate instruments 2.5 to 3.0 mm in diameter without damaging the fragile articular surfaces.

The traction is applied through fingertraps placed on two or three digits. Conventional fingertraps are adequate, but the use of bamboo or fiber fingertraps has caused occasional complaints of postoperative PIP joint pain and contusion of the digital nerves. Soft, flexible nylon fingertraps are ideally suited for the application of traction to the digits and appear to be completely atraumatic (Fig. 3-1).

Joint traction is best applied with a Traction Tower (Concept, Largo, FL), which is designed specifically for wrist arthroscopy. This device measures the applied traction on a spring gauge and maintains the extremity in a stable vertical position (Fig. 3-2). It can be completely sterilized and allows intraoperative positioning of the wrist in varying degrees of flexion and extension, and radial or ulnar deviation.

Without the Traction Tower, joint distraction can be applied through a system of weights, lines, and pulleys in various overhead arrangements (Fig. 3-3). Countertraction about the upper arm and forearm braces can be added to stabilize the extremity, but is more cumbersome than the Traction Tower.

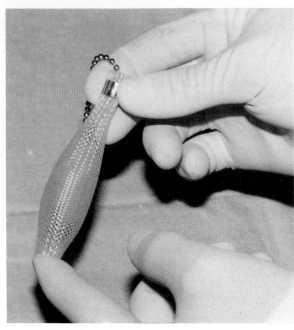

FIGURE 3–1.
Nylon fingertraps are disposable, soft, and flexible. They are provided with a ball, chain, and hook crimped to the distal end. (Concept, Largo, FL.)

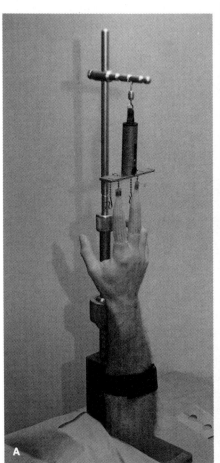

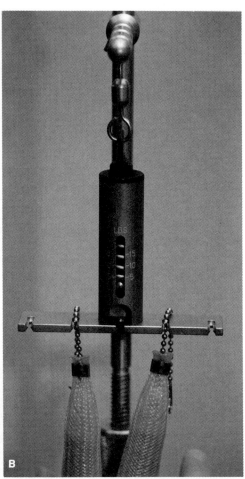

FIGURE 3–2.
(**A**) Complete Traction Tower assembly with fingertraps on index and long fingers. This assembly can be completely sterilized. (**B**) Traction Tower spreader bar and traction scale. The fingertrap chains are attached to slots in the spreader bar. The calibrated spring scale indicates distraction force in pounds.

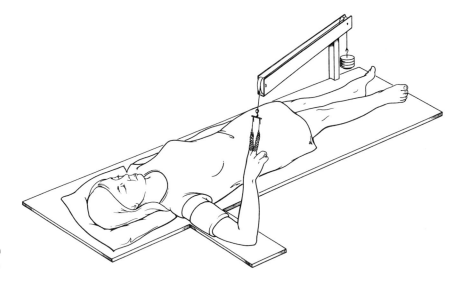

FIGURE 3–3.
Traction assembly using suspension boom and pulleys with counterweights.

IRRIGATION

As in other joints, lactated Ringer's solution is well-suited for irrigation of the wrist during arthroscopic procedures. It is physiologically compatible with the articular cartilage and is rapidly reabsorbed if extravasated from the joint. Other solutions may also be suitable, such as glycine or normal saline. Rarely is more than 500 ml required to complete an entire case. Because the wrist joint capsule is relatively thin and the subcutaneous areolar tissue overlying the wrist dorsally is not dense, distention of the wrist with gas for arthroscopic procedures is impractical.

Infusion pumps have been used successfully for arthroscopic surgery of the wrist. A pump designed to monitor both pressure and flow is capable of safely maintaining an adequate perfusion of the joint, and is especially helpful when suction instruments are used in the wrist (Fig. 3-4). However, the wrist is a small joint and requires only a few milliliters of irrigation solution to maintain adequate distention. Using a patent inflow cannula with at least a 16-gauge bore, gravity-fed inflow is sufficient in almost all cases (Fig. 3-5). Irrigation lines equipped with a small pinch chamber allow an additional 2 to 3 ml of fluid to be pumped into the joint quickly and conveniently when needed. These pinch pump in-fusion lines are presterilized and disposable, and we routinely use them for wrist arthroscopy (Fig. 3-6).

ARTHROSCOPES

Since 1970, several optical designs have been incorporated into arthroscopes; however, the Hopkins rod lens remains the gold standard for arthroscopes of all sizes. Fiberoptic technology continues to improve, and high-quality flexible arthroscopes may eventually become available. However, the recent improvements in very small-diameter rigid arthroscopes makes them well-suited for wrist arthroscopy.

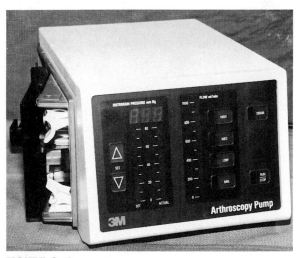

FIGURE 3–4.
Arthroscopy pump for assisted positive-pressure inflow (3M, Minneapolis, MN).

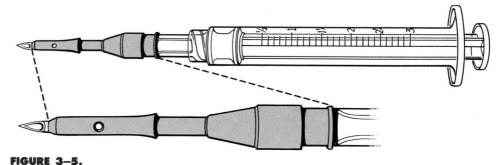

FIGURE 3–5.

Plastic 16-gauge inflow cannula provided with needle and 3-ml syringe for ease of insertion. The collar on the shank of the cannula retains its position in soft tissue. (Concept, Largo, FL.)

Most wrists can be safely distracted enough to accommodate arthroscopes and arthroscope sheaths up to 3 mm in diameter. Larger instruments are difficult to maneuver inside the joint without significant risk of scuffing the fragile hyaline cartilage surface. Children and petite individuals may require even smaller diameter arthroscopes to examine the joint thoroughly, but rarely is an arthroscope smaller than 1.9 mm in outer diameter needed. The fragility of smaller diameter arthroscopes is an economic factor that must be taken into consideration.

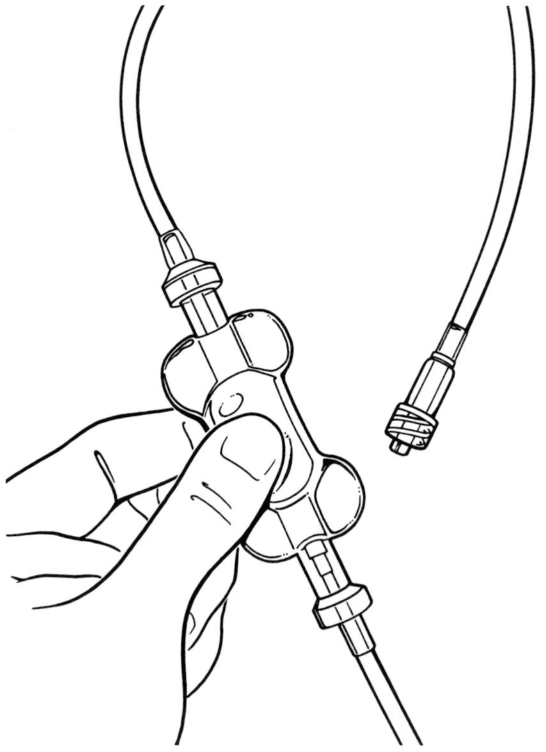

For use in the wrist, the shaft of an arthroscope needs to be only 5 to 10 cm in length. The use of longer instruments in such a superficial joint places a bending fulcrum close to the tip of the arthroscope with considerable leverage on the long extraarticular shaft. This increases the risk of bending or breaking arthroscopes of small diameter and is more awkward and tiring for the surgeon (Fig. 3-7).

To see around the convex surfaces of the proximal row, the distal pole of the scaphoid, and the head of the capitate, a 25° to 30° oblique lens on the tip of the arthroscope is usually necessary. Larger angled lenses are occasionally required to see small recesses such as the opening to the pisotriquetral articulation, but rarely would a smaller angle or straight arthroscope be preferable.

The best arthroscopes have a zero to infinity focal length. They can provide a clear image when tissue is pressed close to the objective lens of the arthroscope inside the joint, while giving equally clear images of objects in the distance.

The arthroscope sheaths are generally used as conduits for inflow or outflow of irrigation solution. They must provide sufficient space between the inside diameter of the sheath and the outside of the arthroscope for the necessary flow of fluid (Fig. 3-8). Smaller tolerances are acceptable when a positive pressure inflow pump is used. However, there should always be enough space for passive flow of irrigation solution through the sheath around the arthroscope when the irrigation solution is elevated 20° to 30°

FIGURE 3–6.

Pinch pump chamber on inflow line with a capacity of 3 ml. (Concept, Largo, FL.)

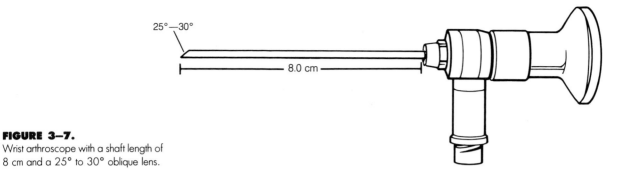

FIGURE 3–7.
Wrist arthroscope with a shaft length of 8 cm and a 25° to 30° oblique lens.

above the wrist. This will ensure that the arthroscope sheath can be used for passive outflow of fluids, even when passive inflow is used through a separate portal.

The design of the distal tip of the arthroscope sheath is a crucial consideration. The distal opening of the sheath must be radiused to avoid accidental scuffing of the articular cartilage. This radiusing should also gently blend with the outside diameter of the sheath obturators to allow gentle insertion through the joint capsule without tearing the synovium.

The sheath should be 1 to 2 mm shorter than the arthroscope when fully seated and locked in place. For arthroscopes with lens angles greater than 30°, it may be necessary to use a sheath with a slightly angled opening so that there is no obstruction of the full field of view. The proximal end of the sheath should have a quick and secure connecting mechanism to accept the trocar or arthroscope. This will allow easy insertion and removal of the

arthroscope from the sheath during the course of a procedure without fumbling to secure the connection.

VIDEO CAMERAS AND COUPLERS

There are a few mandatory specifications for video cameras used in wrist arthroscopy. Most modern video cameras use a small chip sensor with excellent light sensitivity nearly equal to that of tube cameras. The advantage of the chip camera is its lighter weight and smaller size. Short cameras place less leverage on the fragile optics of the small diameter arthroscopes, and cameras are available with 450 to 700 lines of resolution. As the smaller diameter arthroscopes create a small-diameter image, magnifying this image on the video screen will produce a grainy picture unless the camera has high resolution capability.

Ideally, the power source for the video camera

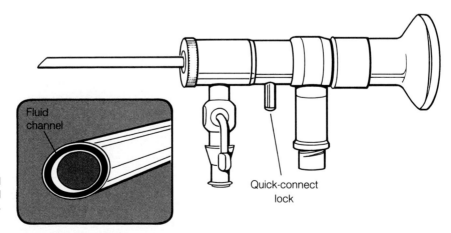

FIGURE 3–8.
Assembled wrist arthroscope and sheath. Note the fluid channel around the outer diameter of the telescope (*inset*).

should have an automatic gain control with quick response to provide optimal brightness for the image in low light situations and protection for the sensitive chip when bright glare is produced by reflection from the white articular surfaces. It should also allow simple correction of red, green, and blue hues for optimal contrast and color reproduction.

The camera cord must be durable but not too stiff or heavy, or the cord may produce a drag on the free movement of the camera. The prongs on the plug connector between the camera cord and the camera power source must also be durable and corrosion resistant. The signal from some cameras is distorted if there is any moisture on these prongs. Larger plugs space the prongs farther apart and obviate this problem.

Some cameras couple directly to the arthroscope lens train without an intervening eyepiece (Fig. 3-9). This system provides certain distinct advantages but also introduces some inherent disadvantages. The direct-connection videoscopes are generally shorter than an assembly using a conventional arthroscope with eyepiece, lens coupler, and video camera. They also eliminate an air space between the coupler and arthroscope lens, reducing moisture condensation and fogging. However, it is less convenient to change arthroscopes when a different lens angle is required or when a smaller diameter arthroscope is necessary to see remote or extremely narrow spaces.

More conventional arthroscopes with an eyepiece mate to the camera by means of a quick-connect coupler that screws onto the camera (Fig. 3-10). These couplers should be vented to minimize moisture condensation on the lenses. Couplers are available in a variety of sizes. As noted earlier, the smaller diameter arthroscopes produce a smaller diameter image that must be magnified. To optimize the image, one must achieve an appropriate balance between size and sharpness. Less light spread over a larger field of view dulls the image. Cameras or monitors with fewer lines of resolution or dots per inch will also produce a less clear image if overly magnified. However, brightly illuminated images improved by high resolution cameras on high resolution monitors can be magnified with good clarity, sharpness, and color resolution.

The degree of magnification is a function of the lens system and the coupler. The coupler is essentially a teleconvertor that zooms in on the image presented by the ocular lens of the arthroscope. Thus, larger coupler lenses produce a larger diameter screen image. Some experimentation with different combinations of arthroscope, camera, and coupler is advisable before deciding on preferences and purchases.

VIDEO MONITORS

The video monitor is a crucial piece of equipment for wrist arthroscopy. Medical-grade monitors are available with up to 750 lines of resolution, providing a large number of pixels on the viewing screen. The greater number of pixels maintains sharper lines of curvature and greater resolution of margins within an image. The monitor should allow convenient and broad spectrum color and tint adjustment with convenient control locations. Glare-free screens are a great advantage because a conventional screen may reflect ceiling lights, radiograph view boxes, and operating room lights and compromise the view of either the surgeon or the assistant.

Finally, the weight and size of the monitor may be a critical consideration, depending on whether it is to be suspended over the patient or placed in a cabinet with limited space. With all of these considerations, the surgeon should play an active role

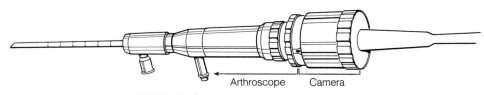

Arthroscope   Camera

FIGURE 3—9.
The video arthroscope connects directly to the camera.

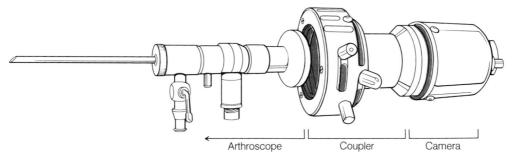

FIGURE 3–10.
Conventional arthroscope with coupler attached to miniature camera.

DOCUMENTATION

The need for documentation of wrist arthroscopy is no different than for arthroscopy of any other joint. There appears to be an increasing need for graphic documentation of pathology and surgical accomplishment in an increasingly litigious society. Documentation also facilitates communication among physicians as well as between physician and patient. The doctor's individual need for documentation should determine the level of investment made for this purpose. Any doctor can draw for the record a graphic representation of the pathology encountered in the wrist and the surgical treatment accomplished, and it is a good practice to do so whether for reference or recollection. Still-frame photography may be more accurate, but is also considerably more expensive and inconvenient. Direct photography through the arthroscope produces the best possible still-frame documentation of intraarticular anatomy. Unfortunately, it may require disconnection of the video camera and articulation of the still-frame camera to the arthroscope. To capture the pathology and the procedure, such a system requires breaking down the video system several times during the course of the procedure. To compose a photograph by means of through-the-lens viewing places the surgeon's face undesirably close to the sterile field. Moreover, the camera can only be adequately sterilized by gassing. This is not only ex-

pensive and time-consuming, but it also makes the camera available for only one case per day. Covering the camera with a sterile drape makes it all the more difficult for through-the-lens viewing and potentially contaminates the eyepiece of the telescope. Still-frame photography directly through the arthroscope is completely impossible if one uses videoscope systems.

Redesigned couplers are being developed to provide a means of docking a 35-mm camera with the coupler without disconnecting the video camera (Fig. 3-11). This system eliminates the need for through-the-lens viewing and camera sterilization. However, the new coupler design lengthens the

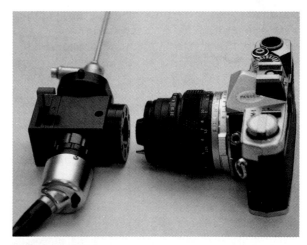

FIGURE 3–11.
The photocoupler attaches the conventional arthroscope to a miniature camera. The red lever relays the composed image laterally to a 35-mm camera for direct image photography. (Prototype, courtesy of Smith and Nephew Dyonics, Andover, MA.)

overall arthroscope–coupler–camera assembly by 2 to 3 cm, which is a slight compromise.

Systems are also available for photographing the image on the screen of the video monitor. This system produces an image composed of pixels on the cathode ray tube (CRT) and is more convenient than direct photography through the arthroscope. These images are perfectly adequate for reference or recall, but they are considerably less clear than images created by direct photography through the arthroscope.

Finally, one can document still-frame representations of various portions of a procedure by picture reproductions of digitized images from the video camera. Video printers are available that can scan and store a video image of higher resolution than that displayed on the video monitor. This image is reproduced in front of a camera that photographs and prints a reproduction. Some of these systems can produce either prints or slides. These relatively expensive systems produce a reasonably clear image, although the image is not nearly as sharp as that achieved by direct photography.

Videotape documentation is a relatively simple procedure. A videocassette recorder connected to the camera or the monitor can be controlled remotely to edit a video summary of the case from start to finish. The case can be recorded on ¾- or ½-inch tape or on the newer ¼-inch tape. The most expensive tape is ¾-inch; it produces by far the best image and can be edited or reproduced through several generations without losing much clarity. Super VHS systems have improved the image quality and reproducibility of ½-inch videotape documentation. The ½-inch videocassette players are more prevalent in homes and offices than the ¾-inch formats, and make review of the tapes more convenient. The newer ¼-inch cassettes accommodate less signal than the other tapes, and therefore retain a less clear but still reasonably acceptable first generation image. They have the distinct advantage of requiring less storage space; approximately ten ¼-inch tapes can be stored in the same space required for one ¾-inch cassette. Again, depending on the individual doctor's documentation needs, this may be an acceptable compromise if reproduction beyond the first generation of recording is not required.

There are three distinct disadvantages to routine videotape documentation of wrist arthroscopy in comparison to still-frame photography. First, review of the images is instrument-dependent. One cannot review the videotape without having available a cassette player and monitor, which considerably limits affordability. Second, it is difficult to access quickly a certain portion of the procedure on videotape because the tape must be reviewed from start to finish, whereas still-frame images can be sorted quickly by hand. Finally, storage of the videotape requires a considerable amount of additional space, and the tapes cannot be readily incorporated into the patient's record.

The doctor must carefully review the need for documentation of surgical procedures before choosing the instrument to be used. Documentation should be purposeful, and the cost and convenience of the system must be a factor in the selection.

ACCESSORY INSTRUMENTS

Probes

Additional information can be obtained from an arthroscopic examination of the wrist by using a small rigid probe used to palpate the surfaces and recesses of intraarticular structures (Fig. 3-12). The probe should be only 1½ mm in diameter to access areas the larger arthroscope cannot reach. An angled tip permits exploration of the joint by retracting veils of soft tissue. More rigid probes provide better tactile sensation and appreciation of tissue consistency and resistance.

The use of a probe in the wrist requires very fine motor skills. It should be manipulated with the thumb and the index or long finger. The extraarticular portion of the probe should have an expanded diameter to allow gentle rotation and manipulation with minimal effort. Simple as it is, the probe is the most important accessory instrument and is used more frequently than any other.

Dissectors

At times, considerable force may be necessary to elevate bone fragments or to wedge open the space between carpals. Probes may not be strong enough for this purpose. A small gently curved or tapered dissector or elevator is most helpful in these circum-

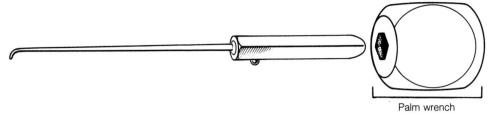

FIGURE 3-12.
Miniature hook probe. A palm wrench improves grip to facilitate instrument insertion. The wrench is removed for tissue manipulation.

stances (Fig. 3-13). The rigidity of the instrument is of utmost importance.

Graspers

To remove loose tissue fragments or to avulse tags of cartilage synovium or ligament that are almost loose, strong grasping forceps are used. For use in the wrist, the optimal diameter of these instruments is approximately 2.5 to 2.75 mm. Of the several jaw designs available I prefer two styles: a flat, tapered jaw with teeth for holding smaller flaps of tissue that are thin or soft, and a rounded and cupped jaw for holding larger fragments of firm tissue such as bone crumbs or fragments of triangular fibrocartilage (TFC; Fig. 3-14).

Smaller instruments are relatively fragile, and moving parts are prone to breakage within the joint. The design of hinge mechanisms at the tip of these instruments is crucial. Hinge pins or pivot points must be precisely machined and thoroughly passivated to resist wear and corrosion. The upper and lower jaws of these instruments should meet with precision. Grasping forceps and other instruments with moving parts should be regularly inspected with magnification to identify fatigue fractures or other defects that indicate potential malfunction or breakage.

The length of grasping forceps and other manually activated instruments is also important. A short

length allows better balance and greater shaft rigidity for small-diameter instruments. Shorter instruments also place finger control nearer the tip of the instrument, improving dexterity. It should rarely be necessary for manually activated wrist instruments to exceed 10 or 12 cm in length.

CUTTING INSTRUMENTS

Trimming, shaping, or excising different tissues within the wrist requires a variety of cutting instruments. Instrument designs for hard tissues differ from those most effective for soft tissue. The angle of surgical approach will influence the choice of instrument. Manually powered cutting instruments commonly used in the wrist consist of curettes, surgical knives, baskets, and punch forceps. Punch forceps are available with suction applied through the shaft for evacuation of cut tissue fragments.

Curettes are used primarily for trimming edges

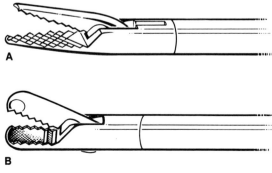

FIGURE 3-14.
(A) The mosquito-tip grasping forceps has fine teeth and is used primarily for soft tissue. **(B)** The cupped-jaw grasping forceps is used primarily for loose bodies and larger tissue fragments.

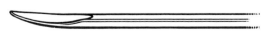

FIGURE 3-13.
A gently curved dissector is stronger than the hook probe for manipulating and disimpacting bone fragments.

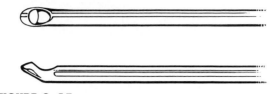

FIGURE 3—15.
Open ring curette with angled tip.

of articular cartilage and for scraping loose soft tissues such as a fibrin clot. They may be of open-ring or closed-cup design and should be constructed of rigid materials to resist bending (Fig. 3-15).

Surgical knives for the wrist are 2 to 3 mm wide and should be razor sharp. The best configuration of the cutting tip is mostly a matter of the surgeon's preference. The most commonly used designs are a curved, double-edged banana blade and a hook blade that cuts in retrograde fashion (Fig. 3-16). Probes and dissecting surgical knives should be of rigid construction and should have expanded extraarticular handles to improve fingertip control.

Basket forceps are available in a variety of tip designs: straight, angled up or down, angled right or left, and scooped or blunt lower jaw (Fig. 3-17). The movable upper jaw may range from 0.5 to 2.5 mm in width. Upper-jaw designs may be hooked or serrated. All of the available configurations notwithstanding, the single most important factor contributing to effective cutting action is the precision with which the upper jaw fits into the lower jaw. Basket forceps cut with a shearing action between the two jaws. If the clearance is too great, clean cuts are not possible and tissue is torn rather than cut.

The suction punch forceps is particularly con-

venient for use in the wrist. It cuts by pinching tissue against the platform of the lower jaw (Fig. 3-18). When the upper jaw is again opened, cut tissue fragments are aspirated through the hollow shaft of the instrument. The added suction capability helps keep the visual field clear and ensure removal of all loose tissue fragments. Moreover, the blunt design of the lower jaw permits cutting tissue close to the joint capsule or bone surface.

Power Instruments

For many cutting tasks in the wrist, power instruments afford an advantage over manually activated instruments. To excise larger volumes of tissue, the

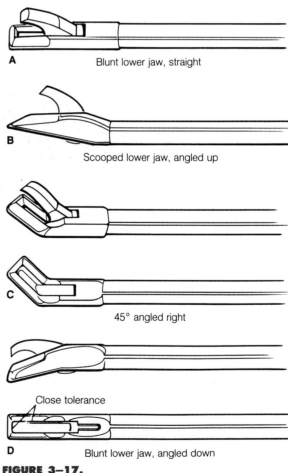

A Blunt lower jaw, straight

B Scooped lower jaw, angled up

C 45° angled right

Close tolerance

D Blunt lower jaw, angled down

FIGURE 3—17.
Arthroscopy basket forceps, straight and angled designs, with blunt or scooped lower jaws. Note the extremely precise tolerance between the upper and lower jaw for precision cuts.

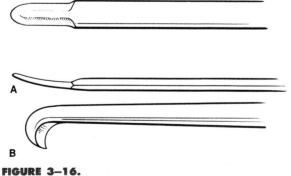

A

B

FIGURE 3—16.
Common arthroscopy knife blade designs. (**A**) Front and side views of a banana blade. (**B**) Retrograde hook blade.

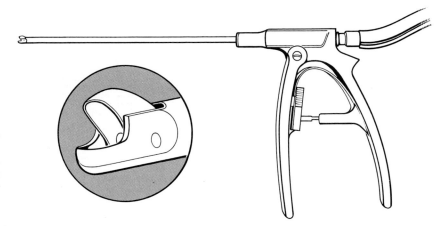

FIGURE 3–18.
Suction punch. Morselized tissue bits are evacuated by wall suction through the tissue trap. Magnified view of cutting tip (*inset*). Note the fine hinge pins protected by action stops on the handle of the punch. (Smith and Nephew Dyonics, Andover, MA.)

rapidly repeating cutting action of a power shaver is much faster. These instruments generally do not cut with the same precision as manually activated instruments. This is of little consequence because the automated action provides so many more cutting passes at the target tissue.

There are numerous tip designs for power instruments. Most employ a rotating blade within a fixed external sheath. The blade cuts against the edges of one or more openings at the tip of the sheath. Depending on the blade and sheath opening design, different power instruments will perform optimally at various rotating speeds (Fig. 3-19). The highest speeds are attainable with pneumatic-driven turbine motors. Speeds in the range of 500 rpm are easily achieved with electric motors.

The size of the window or opening in the external sheath and the speed of the rotating blade limit the size of the tissue fragment cut with each revolution of the blade. Because most power instruments are equipped with suction evacuation for cut tissue fragments, selecting an appropriately sized chip is crucial to prevent clogging of the aspiration channel (Fig. 3-20).

Abrading or excising hard bone fragments in the joint is done best with a power burr. The design of the burr is no less important for the surgeon than it is for a carpenter or jeweler. Coarser cuts for rough large-volume work are made by burrs with fewer and deeper flutes. Fine polishing work is best performed by the burrs that have shallower flutes with less severe angles of approach to the bone surface (Fig. 3-21). Higher speeds of revolution stabilize the burr and reduce shatter but also increase heat production at the cutting surface. Practice is required to use the various burr designs most effectively.

Aside from power supply design (pneumatic or electrical), other important design considerations for the handpiece of power instruments are length, weight, and balance. Heavy or unbalanced handpieces contribute to surgeon fatigue when precision control is essential. Longer instruments increase the bending moment on small-diameter cutting shafts

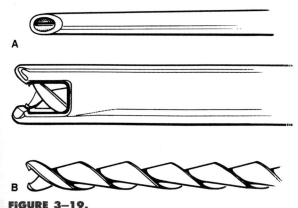

FIGURE 3–19.
Miniature power shaver tip designs. (**A**) Full radius resector. Note the hollow blade within the windowed sheath design. (**B**) High-speed cartilage cutter. (Baxter Edwards, Irvine, CA.)

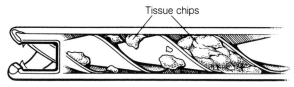

Tissue chips

FIGURE 3–20.
High-speed cartilage cutter evacuating tissue chips. "Force feeding" will cause large chips to clog flutes of the internal blade.

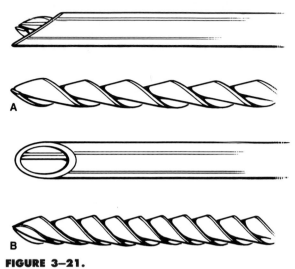

FIGURE 3–21.
(**A**) Coarse cutting burr with deep flutes. (**B**) Fine cutting burr with shallow flutes.

and may bind the internal rotating member or increase heat production at the level of the skin or joint capsule. Although these considerations may seem trivial, they contribute significantly to the success of surgical procedures in the wrist. The surgeon's evaluation of and preferences for manual and power instruments is of great importance.

The precise control of suction at the tip of power instruments remains an unsolved problem. Hospital vacuum systems vary in intensity and sensitivity. Regulators provide gross control of negative pressures and are usually located at a considerable distance from the surgical field. The negative pressure builds through tissue chambers and fluid reservoirs that may be rigid or flexible, and the vacuum is applied through flexible wall tubing. All these factors modulate the suction pressure at the tip of power instruments and can compromise the instrument's effectiveness.

Vent mechanisms have been incorporated into some power instrument designs to place some regulation of suction at the surgeon's fingertips. Consideration should be given to whether these controls require one or two hand operations, and through what range of pressures they are effective. These decisions should not be relegated solely to a hospital purchasing agent.

PERSONNEL

Regular training sessions are necessary to educate personnel responsible for cleaning, packaging, sterilizing, and storing these delicate instruments. Instruments should never be dumped together. Rubber or foam lined trays or protective metal racks are well worth their cost to protect instrument tips from dulling and instrument shafts from bending. Because of the fine tolerances between moving parts, all instruments should be inspected regularly under magnification to locate signs of loosening, binding, or metal fatigue.

BIBLIOGRAPHY

Poehling GG. Hand instruments for small joint arthroscopy. Arthroscopy 1988;4(2):126.
Whipple TL. Powered instruments for wrist arthroscopy. Arthroscopy 1988;4(4):290.

4

Operating Room Environment and the Surgical Team

Wrist arthroscopy is a minimally invasive surgical procedure, and most arthroscopic procedures for the wrist can be performed on an outpatient basis. The surprisingly low level of postoperative discomfort and morbidity further reduces the cost and inconvenience to the patient.

OPERATING ROOM

The operating room should be large enough to accommodate the same amount of electronic and video equipment typically used for arthroscopic procedures in the knee or shoulder. The room should be equipped for general or regional anesthesia and for major extremity procedures to permit the surgeon to respond to any unexpected contingencies that might develop intraoperatively.

The small-diameter arthroscopes used for wrist arthroscopy produce such a small image through the ocular lens that video magnification is essential. The video camera power pack, television monitor, and light source are best arranged on a mobile cart or suspended frame positioned on the side of the operating table opposite the involved extremity. An optional video recorder as well as the nonsterile power systems for motorized surgical instruments should be placed on the same cart or frame.

PATIENT PREPARATION

The patient is positioned supine on the operating table with the shoulder abducted 60° to 90° on a narrow hand table or arm board (Fig. 4-1). Wide hand tables require unnecessary reach by the surgeon or assistant and cause fatigue. I prefer a table no more than 16 inches wide. Alternatively, two parallel arm boards affixed to the side of the operating table will suffice. A pneumatic tourniquet should be placed about the arm, and it may be inflated or not inflated according to the surgeon's preference (see Fig. 4-1).

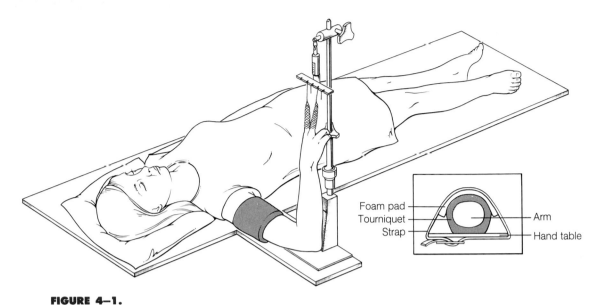

FIGURE 4–1.
The patient is supine on the operating table with the shoulder abducted 60° to 90° and resting on a narrow hand table. A restraining strap encircles the tourniquet and hand table (*inset*).

The wrist should be shaved circumferentially from the midmetacarpals to about 1 inch proximal to the radial styloid. The extremity should be prepped from the tourniquet to the fingertips. The arm is then draped in sterile fashion to expose the extremity distal to the midforearm. I prefer to apply a sterile stockinette rolled above the elbow, and to use an extremity drape with a central hole placed about the arm above the elbow. This leaves the elbow and entire forearm within the sterile surgical field to accommodate any possible surgical procedure, and keeps the folds of the drapes out of the way. The stockinette is cut distally and rolled back to the level of the midforearm, leaving the elbow and most of the forearm covered (Fig. 4-2).

Traction

Traction can be applied to the wrist in a variety of ways. Sterile fingertraps are applied to two or more digits. Wire mesh fingertraps will suffice, but the newer flexible nylon mesh fingertraps cover a larger surface area of the finger and are gentler on the skin (see Fig. 3-1).

There are three common methods of applying traction. The fingertraps can be attached to a sterile line suspended from the ceiling. Weights are then hung from a sling placed about the upper arm over the tourniquet. It is difficult to know precisely how much traction is applied using this method because the hand table absorbs some of the load of the suspended weights. Also it is impossible to move or adjust the operating table without affecting the traction system.

A better system employs a suspension boom such as is used for shoulder arthroscopy. These devices are equipped with pulleys over which a sterile line, attaching to the fingertraps at one end and a weight pan at the other, is passed. The boom is fixed to the side of the operating table, and countertraction is applied by a strap encircling the patient's arm and the hand table together (see Fig. 3-3). This system is adequate but cumbersome to adjust and requires the assistance of circulating nurses in the operating room.

My preferred method of applying traction to the wrist employs a Traction Tower, which can be disassembled for complete sterilization (see Fig. 3-2). The base of the Traction Tower sits on the hand table with a circumferential strap about the patient's upper arm and the hand table. The fingertraps attach to the spreader bar suspended from the top of the tower (see Fig. 4-2). Traction is applied by raising the height of the tower, and it is measured by a spring scale. This system can be easily adjusted to

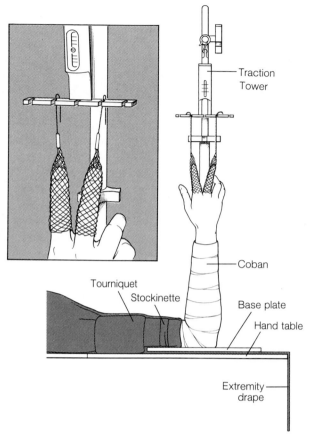

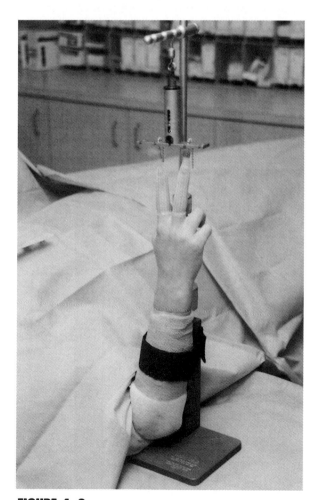

should have a clear view of the video monitor and know how to maneuver the arthroscope to maintain focus in the intraarticular region where the surgeon is working. The assistant should be completely familiar with the operation of all the instruments, including wire drivers, burrs, shavers, and their various attachments. It is sometimes difficult to maneuver the arthroscope and accessory instruments precisely into the required position. These circumstances do not afford the surgeon opportunity to assist with the assembly or adjustment of instruments.

The maintenance of an adequate irrigation system should also be the responsibility of the assistant, who should recognize the need for additional infusion of irrigation solution and should know how to balance the rate of inflow and outflow to avoid

FIGURE 4–2.
The extremity is draped with a stockinette rolled above the elbow and cuffed at the midforearm. A sterile extremity sheet is applied above the elbow and tucked deeply beneath the elbow to accommodate the plate of the Traction Tower. Flexible nylon fingertraps are applied to the index and long fingers with ball chains attached to the spreader bar of the traction scale (*inset*).

FIGURE 4–3.
The Traction Tower is draped into the sterile field. Note the proximal forearm strap for additional security.

position the wrist in flexion, extension, or radial or ulnar deviation, and is much more compact than the other methods (Fig. 4-3).

OPERATING ROOM PERSONNEL

Each member of the surgical team should have defined responsibilities. The surgical assistant or scrub nurse should be familiar with the objectives of the procedure and the instruments to be used. The assistant may be needed to stabilize the arthroscope and camera if both of the surgeon's hands are required for a surgical maneuver. Thus, the assistant intraarticular bleeding or the introduction of bubbles.

Unsterile circulating personnel must be familiar with the operation of all of the video equipment and power instruments, both electric and pneumatic. They should be able to troubleshoot this equipment if a malfunction occurs intraoperatively. The circulating assistant should be responsible for replenishing irrigating solution as required, and for maintaining the appropriate level of negative pressure in the suction system. In addition, the circulating assistant must constantly monitor the tourniquet for any malfunction or spontaneous change of pressure, as well as monitoring the traction system if weights or counterweights are used. The circulating assistant should have immediate back-up equipment available in the event of malfunction and should be able to quickly locate and provide any additional instrumentation required to complete a given procedure. Without this coordinated approach to maintaining and monitoring the array of instruments and equipment required for arthroscopic surgery, procedures can easily become frustrating, if not hazardous.

Complex and sophisticated instrumentation requires careful inspection, cleaning, and maintenance between cases. Instrument technicians charged with these responsibilities should know how the instruments are assembled and how they function. They must ensure that fragile instruments are handled and stored with adequate protection against damage, and that moving parts are regularly inspected, using magnification to identify metal fatigue, corrosion, or other damage. Proper handling and lubrication of instruments will greatly prolong their service life and reliability.

The operating room should be arranged to provide ample room for the surgeon to sit adjacent to the head of the table facing the dorsum of the patient's hand. The assistant should either sit opposite the surgeon, facing the patient's palm, or beside the surgeon at the end of the hand table. The preferred position depends on the assistant's role in handling instruments within the joint. However, the assistant must always have a clear view of the video monitor (Fig. 4-4). The surgeon and assistant should remain comfortable throughout the sometimes tedious procedures. Some will prefer to stand, whereas others will prefer to sit. Stools should have a foot-operated hydraulic height adjustment. Some surgeons prefer arm rests as well. To afford adequate working room

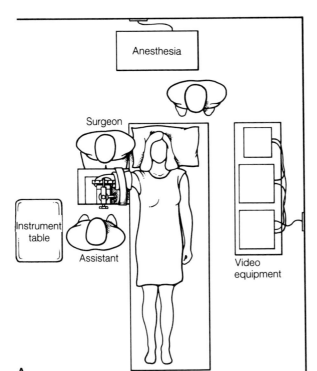

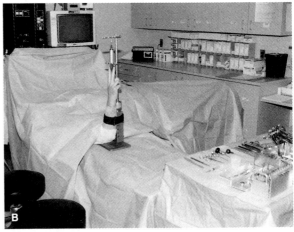

FIGURE 4–4.

(**A**) Operating room arrangement. (**B**) Photograph of operating room set-up with extremity properly draped.

Table 4—1.
SUMMARY OF SURGICAL TEAM RESPONSIBILITIES

Circulating Nurses or Room Assistants

These persons are important to the efficiency of the surgical procedure. They should therefore be familiar with the objectives and techniques of the planned surgical procedure. Responsibilities include the following:

- Maintain the surgical environment.
- Provide for patient comfort and safety.
- Ensure inventory control of disposable supplies.
- Ensure accurate labeling and storage of instruments.
- Ensure that worn or broken instruments are quickly repaired or replaced.
- Ensure the availabiity of instruments, implants, and equipment for the planned procedure and for any contingencies.
- Review equipment and instrument needs with surgeon preoperatively.
- Maintain and operate video equipment and power sources.
- Replace irrigation solution and regulate suction pressure.
- Monitor progress of the procedure and anticipate equipment needs.

Scrub Nurse or Surgical Assistant

This person's primary responsibility is to facilitate the execution of the surgical procedure. Responsibilities include the following:

- Understand the objective and technique for each procedure.
- Organize all sterile instruments and cords in the operative field.
- Anticipate each step in the procedure and have the appropriate selection of sterile instruments in hand.
- Steady the arthroscope, camera, and surgical instruments when necessary.
- Provide retraction if necessary and maintain exposure.
- Keep the surgeon's hand free as much as possible.
- Balance the rate of irrigation inflow and outflow to maintain a clear visual field.
- Recognize immediately any complications and be prepared for contingency situations.
- Apply appropriate bandages and splints.

at the head of the table, anesthesia personnel and their equipment should be positioned at the patient's head on the nonoperative side of the table.

All instruments that might be necessary for an operative procedure and for any contingency should be immediately available in the operating room. There should be an ample supply of cutting, grasping, and retracting instruments and probes on the sterile field. The circulating nurse can provide other sterile instruments as the need arises.

As for any technically demanding surgery, a coordinated and dedicated surgical team is imperative for successful and efficient execution of arthroscopic wrist procedures. Time spent caring for and organizing instruments and training and coordinating personnel is a valuable investment. Table 4-1 summarizes the respective responsibilities that should be assumed by circulating nurses or room assistants, and by scrub nurses or surgical assistants.

BIBLIOGRAPHY

Whipple TL, Marotta JJ, Powell JH III. Techniques of wrist arthroscopy. Arthroscopy 1986;2(4):244.

5

Surgical Anatomy

O f all human diarthrodial joints, the wrist has by far the most complicated anatomy. It is really a system of joints or articulations which together permit motion in six directions around three variable axes. Including the metacarpals, there are 15 bones that provide some 45 articular surfaces of the wrist. Few motions at the wrist involve a single articulation. Rather, motion occurs as a symphony of gliding and rolling movements between several articular surfaces to produce ranges of flexion and extension, radial and ulnar deviation, and pronation and supination. It is therefore understandably difficult to distill painful symptoms associated with motion or loading of the wrist down to a single articulation. To attempt to do so requires a thorough understanding of the anatomy and mechanics of the wrist, and a deliberate, if not tedious, clinical examination.

Minimally invasive surgery of the wrist demands an intimate knowledge of topographical anatomy and the landmarks that can be identified by palpation. With practice, these landmarks are sufficient to allow direct surgical approaches to most intraarticular regions of the wrist with precision and confidence. In addition to intraarticular pathology, there are numerous extraarticular causes of wrist pain, swelling, and other dysfunctions that can be best identified by a systematic investigation of the tendons, nerves, and vessels that cross the wrist. These structures include 24 tendons, two major arteries, two mixed nerves, and many cutaneous branches of the radial and ulnar nerves.

The techniques for regional examination of the wrist based on the patient's clinical complaints are discussed in Chapter 2. This chapter describes surgical approaches to the wrist for minimally invasive techniques. In contrast to most anatomy atlases, here the wrist will be approached as the surgeon encounters it, from the outside in, beginning with the skin and topical landmarks and progressing deeper to the intraarticular structures and surfaces.

ARTHROSCOPY PORTALS

There are ten useful portals for arthroscopy: five for the radiocarpal space, three for the midcarpal space, and two for the distal radioulnar joint (DRUJ). There are also two portals for approaching the carpometacarpal (CMC) joint of the thumb. These portals permit access to specific intraarticular regions and pass between nerves, vessels, and tendons. These portals are identified in Table 5-1. With attention to external landmarks, portals can be located reliably and repeatedly. Indeed, one can develop an intuitive sense of internal anatomy, allowing atraumatic insertion of instruments between carpal bones for intraarticular procedures.

LANDMARKS

There are several readily palpable landmarks consisting of prominences, dimples, and bone intervals. Most of these can be identified even in obese or swollen subjects (Fig. 5-1).

The radial styloid is readily palpable in the snuff box and can be followed in a dorsal proximal direction to the edge of the second extensor compartment. Dorsally, Lister's tubercle can be identified easily. The extensor pollicis longus (EPL) angles around the tubercle on its ulnar side. Most of the dorsal margin of the distal radius can be palpated through the second and fourth extensor compartments on either side of Lister's tubercle. Passively extending the wrist reveals the dorsal margin of the distal radius more clearly by reducing the profile of the proximal carpal row (Fig. 5-2).

The interval between the radius and the head of the ulna can also be palpated easily. This interval is best identified with the wrist held in supination, which relaxes the dorsal capsule of the DRUJ. In a more ulnar direction, the ulnar styloid can be felt. The styloid process is most prominent when the wrist is in neutral rotation. When in slight pronation, the distal margin of the ulnar head can be felt.

Distally, the prominence of the base of the first metacarpal can be palpated. It is easiest to identify the base of the first metacarpal with the thumb ab-

Table 5–1.
ARTHROSCOPY PORTALS FOR RADIOCARPAL SPACE

PORTAL	TOPOGRAPHIC LOCATION	UTILITY	INTRAARTICULAR LOCATION
1-2	Between first and second compartments, dorsal aspect of snuff box, immediately adjacent to EPL and ECRL intersection	View dorsal capsule; inflow for ulnar pathology; instrumentation for radial styloidectomy	Dorsal aspect of radial styloid
3-4	Between third and fourth compartments, distal to Lister's tubercle	Primary entry for arthroscope	Immediately above TFCC attachment to radius
4-5	Ulnar to EDC/little	Primary accessory portal for probe	Immediately above TFCC attachment to radius
6-R	Radial to sixth compartment	Arthroscopic view of LT ligament; accessory portal for TFCC procedures	Through dorsal ligamentous portion of TFCC immediately beneath LT ligament
6-U	Ulnar to sixth compartment	Primary inflow portal; best arthroscopic view of UC ligaments	Through prestyloid recess, just over TFCC articular disc

ECRL, extensor carpi radialis longus; EDC, extensor digitorum communis; EPL, extensor pollicis longus; LT, lunotriquetral; TFCC, triangular fibrocartilage complex; UC, ulnocarpal.

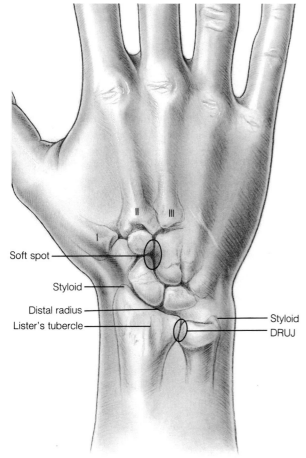

FIGURE 5–1.
Topographical landmarks of the wrist: radial styloid; Lister's tubercle; dorsal margin of the distal radius; interval between radius and head of the ulna; ulnar styloid; base of the first (I), second (II), and third (III) metacarpals, soft spot marking midcarpal space; and the distal radioulnar joint (DRUJ).

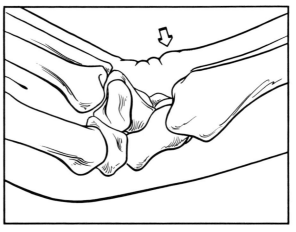

FIGURE 5–2.
Right wrist in dorsiflexion. As the lunate and capitate extend, the distal dorsal margin of the radius becomes more prominent and palpable.

ducted. With reference to a radiograph of the wrist, note the orientation of the first CMC joint; it angles distally toward the base of the second metacarpal. This orientation is important to remember when attempting to inject or instrument the CMC joint of the thumb. The base of the second metacarpal is also prominent and readily palpable, as is the base of the third metacarpal. The CMC joints of the second and third rays are oriented perpendicular to the long axis of the radius.

Midway between the base of the second metacarpal and Lister's tubercle is a soft spot. It can best be felt with the wrist in slight extension. This soft spot marks the level of the midcarpal space. In neu-

tral radioulnar deviation, the midcarpal space is located approximately 8 to 10 mm distal to the dorsal margin of the distal radius, and follows essentially the same contour as the distal radius. In petite subjects, the radius of the curvature of the midcarpal space is less, so this interval appears more curved than in larger subjects.

Tendon landmarks on the wrist can also be identified without difficulty (Fig. 5-3). The first, second, and third extensor compartments mark the boundaries of the anatomical snuff box. It is easy to feel the point of intersection of the second and third extensor compartments, the extensor carpi radialis longus (ECRL), and the EPL, respectively. A straight line drawn from this intersection to Lister's tubercle marks the course of the EPL.

Using a thumbnail ulnar to the EPL, the physician can feel the radial side of the extensor digitorum communis (EDC) tendon to the index finger. This marks the radial margin of the fourth extensor compartment. The ulnar margin of the fourth compartment is similarly identified by the EDC tendon to the little finger, which can be found in a similar manner immediately distal to the interval between the radius and ulna. It is usually not possible to palpate the extensor digiti quinti (EDQ) unless the little finger is actively extended; however, the extensor carpi ulnaris (ECU) tendon in the sixth extensor compartment is always prominent and easy to identify. It is about 6 mm in diameter and can be felt or

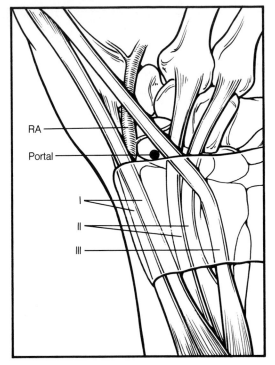

FIGURE 5–3.

Anatomic snuff box. The snuff box is defined by the first (I), second (II), and third (III) extensor compartments. The radial artery (RA) runs in a groove along the volar aspect of the snuff box. There is safe arthroscopic access to the radioscaphoid space in the dorsal aspect of the snuff box.

seen coursing distally from the radial side of the ulnar styloid (Fig. 5-4).

PORTALS

With the wrist in neutral position, the intersections of the above described articular contours and extensor tendon compartments will define the portals for wrist arthroscopy. For the radiocarpal space, the portals are identified by the extensor compartments between which they lie, or to which they relate most closely (see Table 5-1). In the midcarpal space, the portals are less precisely named according to the location where they enter the joint (Table 5-2). Skin punctures for any of these portals should be oriented longitudinally to avoid cutting any of the many branches of cutaneous nerves or dorsal veins. The skin punctures heal spontaneously and can be con-

verted to transverse or longitudinal skin incisions for arthrotomy if necessary.

CUTANEOUS NERVES AND DORSAL VEINS

In the vicinity of all of the arthroscopy portals lie the arborizations of the dorsal cutaneous branches of the radial and ulnar nerves. Although the locations of these cutaneous branches are variable, the radial cutaneous nerve is usually located in close approximation to the intersection of the second and third extensor compartments. This nerve arborizes immediately proximal to this point and usually has at least three main branches (Fig. 5-5). The dorsal cutaneous branch of the ulnar nerve courses superficially around the ulna from the volar to the dorsal aspect. It becomes a dorsal structure at some variable level between the triquetrum and the junction of the middle and distal thirds of the ulna. Most commonly, however, it presents dorsally about two fingerbreadths proximal to the ulnar styloid. Typically, it has fewer branches than the radial cutaneous nerve.

Dorsal veins generally have a longitudinal orientation and are highly variable in number. They are fairly mobile in subcutaneous tissue and can be easily displaced from side to side. Dorsal veins are vulnerable to scalpel laceration, but the introduction of blunt or tapered instruments usually displaces the dorsal veins without injury.

DORSAL RETINACULA

The principal dorsal retinaculum is approximately 2 cm in width and is composed of dense fibers running obliquely across the distal radius and ulna (Fig. 5-6*A*). It overlies all 12 extensor tendons and divides them into respective compartments by means of vertical septae that insert on the radius, the ulna, or the dorsal capsule of the distal radioulnar joint. The dorsal retinaculum maintains the close approximation of the extensor tendons to the bone and prevents bow stringing in wrist extension. The vertical septae maintain the respective positions of the extensor tendons during radial and ulnar deviation of the wrist to provide each tendon group with its best mechanical advantage.

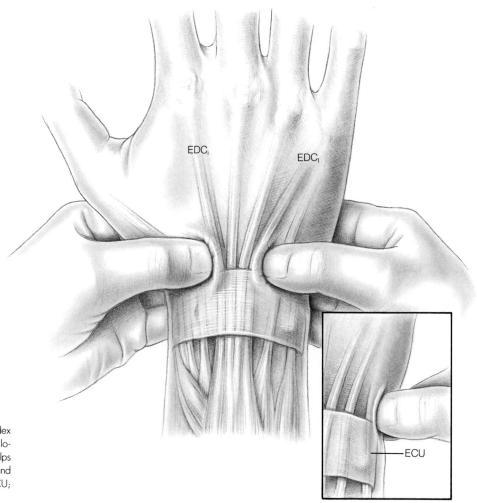

FIGURE 5–4.
Extensor digitorum communis to the index (EDC$_i$) and little fingers (EDC$_l$) can be located with thumbnail pressure. This helps to identify the location of the 3-4 and 4-5 portals. Extensor carpi ulnaris (ECU; inset).

EDC$_i$

EDC$_l$

ECU

Table 5–2.
ARTHROSCOPY PORTALS FOR MIDCARPAL SPACE

PORTAL	TOPOGRAPHIC LOCATION	UTILITY	INTRAARTICULAR LOCATION
RMC	Midway between the base of second MC and dorsal margin of distal radius, in line with radial edge of third MC	Primary arthroscope position for midcarpal space	Scaphocapitate interval proximally
UMC	Same level as RMC, in line with fourth metacarpal	Accessory instruments for midcarpal space	Intersection of CHTL
STT	Ulnar to EPL, in line with radial margin of second MC	Instrumentation of STT joint	Between distal pole of scaphoid, trapezium, and trapezoid

CHTL, capitate, hamate, triquetrum, and lunate; EPL, extensor pollicis longus; MC, metacarpal; RMC, radial midcarpal; STT, scaphotrapeziotrapezoid; UMC, ulnar midcarpal.

supination. The need for this secondary retinaculum for the ECU is apparent when one considers the fact that the primary retinaculum is tight over the ulna in pronation, but loosens in supination (Fig. 5-6*C*). Therefore, the additional structure is required to stabilize the ECU through all degrees of forearm rotation.

Frequently, there is an additional septum within the first extensor compartment separating one of the slips of the extensor pollicis brevis (EPB). This subdivision of the first extensor compartment should always be sought and released when decompressing de Quervain's stenosing tenosynovitis.

CAPSULE AND EXTRINSIC LIGAMENTS

The system of ligaments on the dorsum of the wrist is relatively simple (Fig. 5-7). A condensation of fibers thickens the dorsal capsule. Beginning ulnar to Lister's tubercle, these fibers course distally and ulnarward to insert on the dorsal margins of the lunate and triquetrum. Occasionally, this thickening extends from the lunate distally to the hamate. The floor of the tendon compartment of the EDQ is also thickened. The fibers here run obliquely from the radius to the ulna and blend with the dorsal capsule of the DRUJ. From the distal pole of the scaphoid, running transversely to the triquetrum, is the strong scapho-capito-triquetral ligament. Other than these three discrete thickenings, the remainder of the dorsal wrist capsule is relatively thin and monotonous.

The dorsal capsule arises from the radius 1 to 2 mm proximal to the edge of the articular cartilage. Inside the joint, the synovial membrane arises adjacent to the articular cartilage and reflects over areolar tissue, then adheres to the visceral surface of the capsule. This arrangement provides slight laxity in the dorsal capsule to accommodate wrist flexion. However, there is no evidence of capsule laxity when viewed arthroscopically. In fact, when the dorsal synovium does not course immediately distally from the edge of the articular cartilage, one may reasonably suspect an avulsion injury of the dorsal capsule from the radius. In such cases, 1 or 2 mm of exposed bone not capped by articular carti-

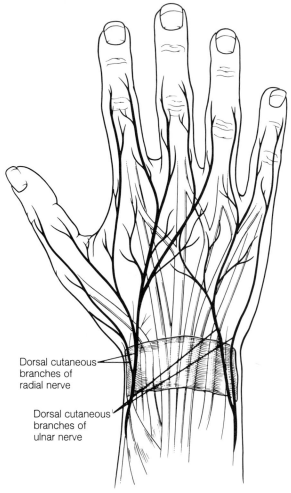

Dorsal cutaneous branches of radial nerve

Dorsal cutaneous branches of ulnar nerve

FIGURE 5–5.

Radial and ulnar cutaneous nerve branches. A branch of the radial sensory nerve is usually in close proximity to the intersection of the extensor carpi radialis longus (ECRL) and extensor pollicis longus (EPL). The ulnar cutaneous nerve has a more variable form and may present dorsally 1 to 5 cm proximal to the ulnar styloid.

On the ulnar side of the wrist, the ECU tendon passes through a separate retinacular sheath deep to the primary dorsal retinaculum (Fig. 5-6*B*). This secondary envelopment of the ECU maintains its position over the head of the ulna. Distally, the tendon inserts on the dorsal aspect of the base of the fifth metacarpal. Therefore, the distal 2 to 3 cm of the tendon traverse a wide excursion from the point of constraint under the secondary retinaculum, as the hand rotates nearly 180° through pronation and

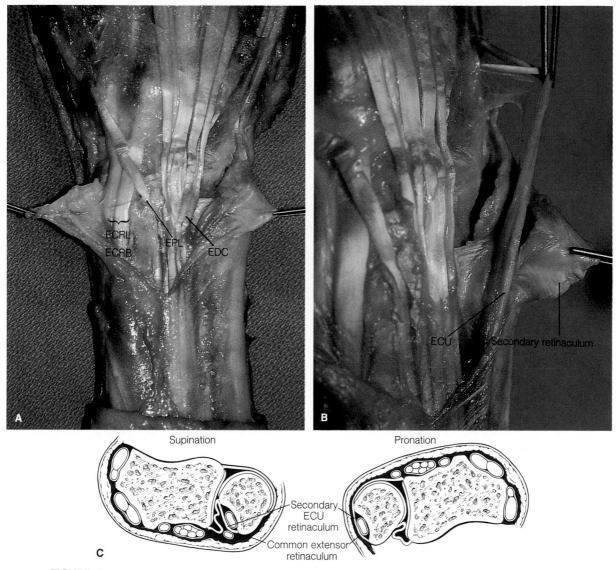

FIGURE 5–6.

Extensor retinacula. (**A**) Right hand dissection. The primary retinaculum has been divided over the fourth extensor compartment, on the extensor digitorum communis (EDC), and retracted. Note the extensor pollicis longus (EPL) crossing the extensor carpi radialis longus (ECRL) and extensor carpi radialis brevis (ECRB). Note the extensor digiti quinti (EDQ) and extensor carpi ulnaris (ECU), still covered by a secondary retinaculum. (**B**) The secondary retinaculum has been opened to expose the ECU contained in a thick tunnel over the head of the ulna. (**C**) The common extensor retinaculum is tight over the ECU in pronation, but loosens in supination. In supination, the secondary ECU retinaculum alone constrains the ECU tendon in its groove.

lage may be seen along the dorsal rim of the radius (Fig. 5-8).

Farther to the ulnar side of the wrist, the same configuration of attachment exists between the articular disc of the triangular fibrocartilage (TFC),

the dorsal synovium, and the dorsal capsule, here composed of the floor of the fifth and sixth extensor compartments. Immediately proximal to the dorsal edge of the fibrocartilage, the dorsal capsule of the distal radioulnar joint separates from the floor of the

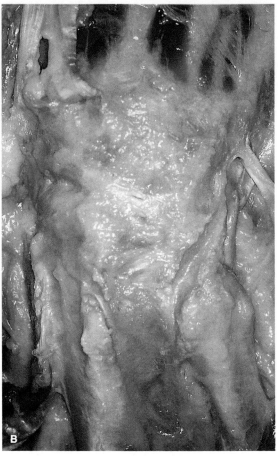

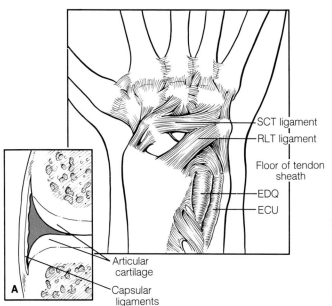

FIGURE 5–7.

Dorsal capsular ligaments. (**A**) Schematic of primary dorsal ligaments. The extensor digiti quinti (EDQ) and the extensor carpi ulnaris (ECU) tendon sheaths have transverse fibers proximally that reinforce the capsule of the distal radioulnar joint and give rise to oblique longitudinal fibers that insert on the dorsal rim of the lunate and triquetrum. Schematic of juxtaarticular synovial attachment (*inset*). Note the attachment of the capsular ligaments proximal and distal to the synovial attachment. This arrangement limits the size of the synovial space, even when the joint capsule is lax in extended positions. (**B**) The dissection of dorsal capsular ligaments in the right wrist. Note the presence of the transverse scapho-capito-triquetral (SCT) ligament, the radiolunotriquetral (RLT) ligament, and the floors of the EDQ and ECU tendon sheaths. The ECU has been retracted toward the ulna.

extensor compartments. It attaches along an oblique line on the ulna metaphysis (Fig. 5-9). The DRUJ dorsal capsule becomes taut in pronation but is little affected by wrist flexion.

The proximal carpal row accommodates attachment of the dorsal capsule along a narrow rim that extends obliquely across the waist of the scaphoid. It continues across the thin dorsal edge of the lunate and the distal dorsal edge of the triquetrum. This narrow attachment completes the dorsal enclosure of the radiocarpal space.

There are no collateral ligaments of the wrist per se. Bowers has correctly noted that an ulnar collateral ligament attaching anywhere on the carpus would inhibit pronation and supination as the wrist rotates about the stationary ulna.* In fact, no semblance of ligamentous structure has been found ulnar to the floor of the ECU compartment. On the con-

---

* Bowers WH, *personal communication, June 1988.*

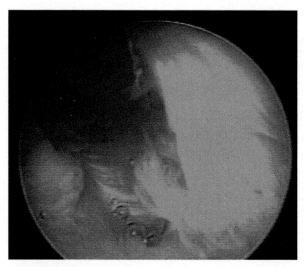

FIGURE 5–8.

The dorsal capsule avulsed from distal radius, viewed from the 1-2 portal of the right wrist. Note the disruption of capsule fibers in the center image; raw bone represents the exposed dorsal rim of the radius (between 6 and 9 o'clock).

trary, the wrist capsule is thin between the extensor and flexor carpi ulnaris tendons and overlies only the prestyloid recess.

Similarly, the capsule is relatively thin on the radial side of the wrist, except for the floor of the first extensor compartment. Coursing distally to the trapezium, this structure may limit ulnar deviation to some extent and thereby function as a radial collateral ligament. No other collateral ligament or capsule thickening can be found in the anatomic snuff box dorsal to the first extensor compartment.

Between the proximal and distal carpal rows, the dorsal capsule remains thin radially but is reinforced on the ulnar side by the continuation of the floor of the ECU compartment. With severe flexion injuries, even this ulnar reinforcement can be avulsed. The midcarpal space then will communicate with the CMC joints of the little or ring fingers. This lesion is uncommon. More often, capsular avulsion injuries are seen on the radial side at the base of the second and third metacarpals where the flexor carpi radialis longus and brevis insert.

On the volar side of the wrist, the supporting ligaments are larger and more extensive, reflecting the quadruped ancestry of humans. Viewed from the palmar surface, the extrinsic ligaments appear flat and unimpressive, but they can be seen to form two arches, one with the apex on the broad flat surface of the lunate, the other with the apex on the body of the capitate (Fig. 5-10). Both arches have similar points of origin—the radial styloid and the anterior aspect of the head of the ulna. The base of the distal arch, however, is wider than that of the proximal arch. The radial leg of the distal arch is the radioscaphocapitate (RSC) ligament. It provides the fulcrum over which the scaphoid flexes with wrist flexion or radial deviation. This ligament may stretch or rupture completely in combination with tears of the scapholunate intrinsic ligament, producing scapholunate dissociation with rotatory subluxation of the scaphoid.

The ulnar leg of the distal arch has three distinct points of attachment. It arises from the fovea in the head of the ulna as the ulnotriquetral (UT) ligament, blending with the volar edge of the triangular fibrocartilage complex (TFCC). This ligament attaches firmly to the broad flat volar surface of the triquetrum. It continues distally across the proximal pole of the hamate to attach finally on the flat volar surface of the body of the capitate. Some of the fibers of this ligament attach to the proximal pole of the hamate. A stronger ligament, however, fans in an ulnar direction from the triquetrum to attach on the

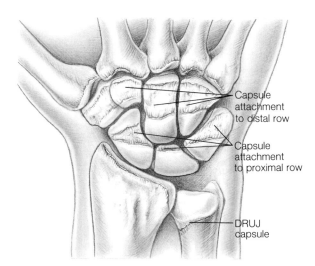

Capsule attachment to distal row

Capsule attachment to proximal row

DRUJ capsule

FIGURE 5–9.

Attachments of dorsal capsular ligaments. Note the oblique line on the ulnar metaphysis representing the attachment of the distal radioulnar joint (DRUJ) capsule (see Fig. 5–7A). Note a narrow line of capsule attachment on the dorsal aspect of the lunate.

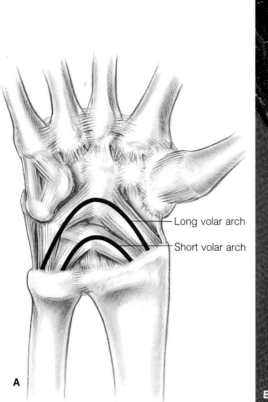

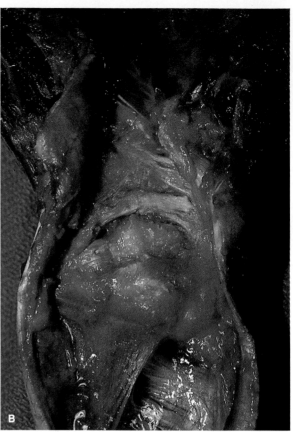

FIGURE 5–10.
Volar extrinsic ligaments. (**A**) Schematic of the volar ligament system depicts two arches with near common points of origin. The long arch centers its apex on the capitate and consists of the ulnotriquetral, triquetro-hamate-capitate, and radioscaphocapitate ligaments. The short arch centers its apex on the lunate and consists of the ulnolunotriquetral and radiolunotriquetral ligaments. Note also the short radioscapholunate ligament (ligament of Testut) within the short arch. (**B**) Volar dissection of the right wrist depicting long and short ligament arches. The prominence beneath the short arch is the lunate in the dorsal intercalary segment instability orientation, seen through the space of Porrier.

hamate on the base of the hook of the hamate. This latter ligament is the strong triquetrohamate ligament that together with the triquetrocapitate ligament provides stability to the midcarpal joint.

The proximal arch has a very low profile and appears slightly longer on the radial side. It is composed of the radiolunotriquetral (RLT) ligament, which arises from the radial styloid and the UT ligament. The radial and ulnar bifurcation of these ligaments is not always readily apparent when viewed from the volar aspect of the joint capsule, but it can be appreciated arthroscopically. The short radioscapholunate (RSL) ligament arising from the

prominent edge of the radius fills in the space bounded by the proximal arch.

These ligaments have a very different appearance from the intraarticular side when viewed arthroscopically. Viewed from within, all of the volar ligaments have higher profiles and stand in relief to the volar capsule (Fig. 5-11). In the radiocarpal space, the ligaments are seen as separate distinct structures. Arising from the radial styloid is the RSC ligament. Immediately ulnar to that structure is the slightly broader RLT ligament, which bifurcates in front of the proximal pole of the scaphoid. Half of this ligament inserts on the broad volar surface of

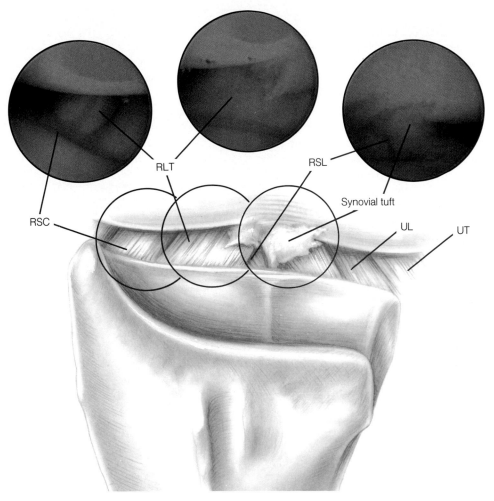

FIGURE 5—11.

The volar radiocarpal ligament of the right wrist. The radiolunotriquetral (RLT) ligament is most prominent centrally; the radioscaphocapitate (RSC) ligament is to the left. The volar synovial tuft (*right*) covers the short radioscapholunate (RSL) ligament of Testut. UL, ulnolunate ligament; UT, ulnotriquetral ligament.

the lunate, and the other half extends almost transversely to reach the triquetrum. These two ligament roots arising from the radial styloid form the radial arms of the distal and proximal ligament arches described above.

Immediately volar to the scapholunate interval internally is a tuft of synovium that extends into the joint from the volar capsule like a salmon-colored plume. This synovial tuft is a consistent structure and a most helpful landmark during arthroscopic examination of the radiocarpal space. It marks the scapholunate interval and the sagittal ridge

between the scaphoid and lunate facets of the radius. Immediately radial to this tuft from the inside of the joint, the short RSL ligament can be seen. This ligament has a much lower profile than the RSC ligament and the RLT ligament, and its fibers run almost perpendicular to the articular surface of the radius. This short but important ligament, known as the ligament of Testut, reinforces the volar capsule and limits extension of the proximal carpal row on the radius.

There is a relatively weak spot in the volar capsule between the RSL ligament and the broad RLT ligament. As evidenced by arthrography, this interval may vary from a potential space to an actual recess extending up to 1 cm proximal to the articular surface of the radius. This is the space of Porrier, into which the lunate may dislocate toward the volar in extension compression injuries.

On the ulnar side of the radiocarpal space, the ulnolunate (UL) and UT ligaments can be seen internally. These ligaments are less prominent than the radiocarpal ligaments. They have a flat profile and bifurcate in front of the triquetrum from their common origin on the ulna. The two resulting ligaments form the ulnar legs of the proximal and distal volar ligament arches described above. Arthroscopically, the bifurcation of these ligaments can be seen best from the 6-U portal, but is sometimes apparent from the 6-R.

INTRINSIC LIGAMENTS

The intrinsic ligaments of the wrist are very short, thin, and sometimes membranous structures that lace the carpal bones together in the proximal and distal carpal rows. The fibers of the ligaments arise from the edges of the carpal bones but blend with the overlying articular cartilage (see Fig. 9-2). There are no intrinsic ligaments within the midcarpal space. Indeed, the midcarpal space is confluent with the scapholunate joint, the lunotriquetral joint, the trapeziotrapezoid joint, the capitotrapezoid joint, and the capitohamate joint (Fig. 5-12). On arthrography, contrast material injected into the midcarpal space should fill each of these five adjoining intervals. The intrinsic ligaments, however, will limit the flow of dye into the radiocarpal space and into the CMC joints.

The scapholunate and lunotriquetral ligaments are the most clinically important of the intrinsic ligaments.[1] Under normal circumstances, they are visible only from the radiocarpal interval (Fig. 5-13). Both of these ligaments are relatively lax under most circumstances. They allow flexion between the scaphoid and the lunate as well as some translation in the sagittal plane between the lunate and triquetrum. They accommodate the normal twisting movement within the proximal carpal row that occurs in extremes of pronation and supination.

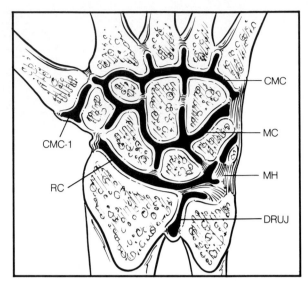

FIGURE 5—12.
The synovial compartments of the wrist. Note that the midcarpal space may communicate with the carpometacarpal space 2-5. Intrinsic carpal ligaments would not be visible arthroscopically in the midcarpal space. CMC, carpometacarpal space; CMC-1, thumb carpometacarpal space; DRUJ, distal radioulnar joint; MC, midcarpal space; MH, meniscus homolog; RC, radiocarpal space.

Under axial load, as in power grip or palmar weight bearing, the intrinsic ligaments become tight. They limit the spread of the proximal carpal row, as the capitate and hamate wedge proximally (Fig. 5-14).

TRIANGULAR FIBROCARTILAGE COMPLEX

Interposed between the proximal row and the distal end of the ulna is the TFCC. This much-studied structure remains poorly understood. It is composed of a central disc of fibrocartilage that merges on its volar edge with the volar ulnocarpal ligaments, and on its dorsal edge with the floors of the EDQ and ECU tendon compartments.

In coronal section, the central disc is generally wedge-shaped. Radially, it inserts on the articular surface of the radius by merging with the hyaline cartilage of the sigmoid notch and the lunate facet (Fig. 5-15). On the ulnar side, the central disc at-

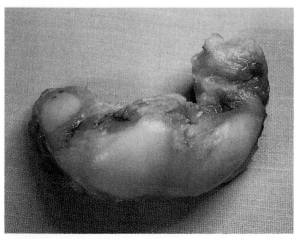

FIGURE 5–13.

Right proximal carpal row. Viewed from the proximal volar aspect, the lunotriquetral and scapholunate intrinsic ligaments blend into the hyaline cartilage of the carpal bones. Note the articular surface for the pisiform on the triquetrum (*far left*).

taches to the base of the ulnar styloid process. The central and radial portions of the disc are avascular, but the peripheral third of this fibrocartilage contains a dense network of capillaries supplied by branches of the ulnar artery (Fig. 5-16). Mechanically, the central disc of the TFCC provides an articular sling for the proximal surface of the triquetrum and the ulnar half of the lunate.

The volar UL and UT ligaments are considered part of the TFCC. They arise from a depression on the volar aspect of the distal surface of the ulna, adjacent to the ulnar styloid (Fig. 5-17). Distally, they insert on the flat volar surfaces of the lunate and triquetrum. These ligaments limit extension and radial deviation. They are tightened in supination, explaining in part why there is less radial deviation in supination than in pronation. The prestyloid recess communicates with the radiocarpal space through an opening in the ulnar aspect of the TFCC.

The vascular peripheral portions of the central disc are thickened dorsally and volarly, and are referred to as distal radioulnar ligaments. In fact, the tensile or ligamentous function of this thickening has not been documented conclusively. Whipple and Martin demonstrated in a cadaver study that cutting these thickened margins of the disc had no effect on the rotational stability of the DRUJ.[2]

The disc is suspended from the joint capsule over the head of the ulna, and sweeps over the ulna like a fan during pronation and supination. With supination, the radius translates dorsally, pulling the TFCC disc with it over the ulna, and tightening the thickened dorsal margin (Fig. 5-18). With full pronation, the opposite occurs; the radius translates slightly toward the volar, pulling the TFCC disc with it and tightening the thick volar margin. Also, as the radius shortens in pronation, the central disc is tightened over the volar aspect of the ulnar head (Fig. 5-19). Interposed between the ulnar head and proximal carpal row, the disc is vulnerable to compression injury when the wrist sustains excessive axial loads.

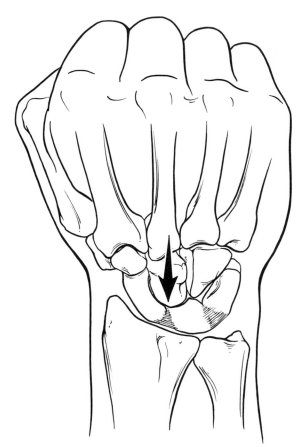

FIGURE 5–14.

The power grip transmits axial force through the capitate and hamate. The proximal carpal row cuts tightly around the capitate and hamate, compressing the distal aspect of the proximal row and spreading its proximal aspect with tension on the intrinsic ligaments.

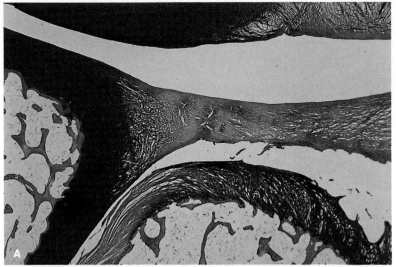

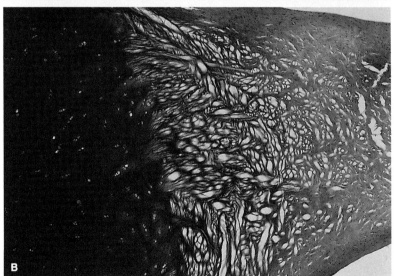

FIGURE 5–15.
Photomicrograph showing triangular fibrocartilage complex central disc attachment to the radius. (**A**) Fibers of the central disc are attached to the distal ulnar corner of the sigmoid notch distal to the head of the ulna. (**B**) Fibrocartilage fibers merge with hyaline cartilage fibers of the articular surface of the radius. (Safranin-O stain; courtesy of B. Mandelbaum, M.D., Santa Monica, CA.)

DISTAL RADIOULNAR JOINT

The DRUJ is a perplexing structure. The mechanical function of this articulation seems simple enough; the radius rotates about the head of the ulna. However, subtle changes in articular contact occur that must be accommodated by the surrounding and supporting soft tissues. When the forearm is fully supinated, the radius appears longer than the ulna at the wrist. In pronation, the radius shortens because it crosses to the medial side of the ulna, assuming an oblique rather than parallel relationship to the ulna.

In this oblique position, the articular surface of the sigmoid notch articulates slightly more proximally with the ulna, and with a more angular orientation to the axis of the forearm. Therefore, the articular surface of the sigmoid notch must slope toward the radial shaft from distal to proximal to accommodate the changing angle of the radius relative to the ulna.

The contact zone on the sigmoid notch makes a dorsal shift in pronation and a volar shift in supination. The movement at this joint through pronation and supination is really a combination of rolling and sliding, with the sliding occurring in

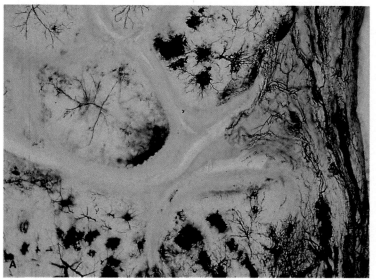

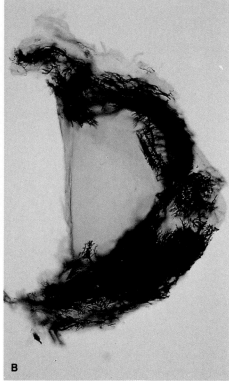

FIGURE 5–16.

Photomicrograph (whole mount) showing the vascular supply to the triangular fibrocartilage complex central disc. India ink injection demonstrates the capillary network in the peripheral one-third of the articular disc. The central two-thirds are avascular. (**A**) Coronal section. (**B**) Transverse section. (India ink; courtesy of S. Arnoczky, D.V.M., Dipl. A.C.V.S., New York, NY.)

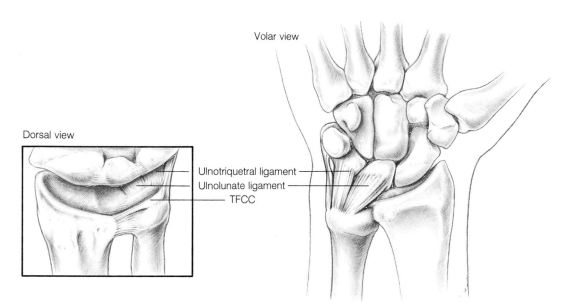

FIGURE 5–17.

The ligamentous portion of the triangular fibrocartilage complex (TFCC). Volar ulnocarpal ligaments arise from a depression in the volar aspect of the ulnar head and merge with the volar margin of the TFCC central disc, continuing distally to insert on the flat volar surfaces of the lunate and triquetrum.

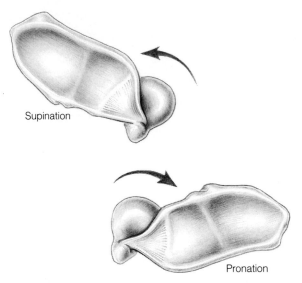

FIGURE 5–18.
Rotational relationship between the radius, ulna, and triangular fibrocartilage complex. In supination, the radius shifts dorsally, tightening the dorsal margin of the central disc. In pronation, the radius shifts volarward, tightening the volar margin of the central disc.

the anteroposterior direction, as well as proximally and distally. Loading forces on this joint may occur axially, coronally, sagittally, or in rotation (Fig. 5-20). Understandably, the soft tissues that stabilize this joint through such complex movements and loads are complicated and must function in harmony.

The most superficial part of the dorsal DRUJ capsule is the floor of the ECU and EDQ tendon sheaths. The fibers in these sheaths are oriented

horizontally, perpendicular to the tendons they support. Immediately proximal to the greatest diameter of the ulnar head, the DRUJ capsule separates from the tendon sheaths, attaching to the dorsal aspects of the radius and ulna along oblique lines that approach the interosseous membrane. Here the DRUJ capsule forms an axilla about 12 to 15 mm proximal to the level of the distal surface of the ulna. The axilla of the capsule is lax in neutral rotation, but is stretched tight in pronation and supination. The volar attachment of the capsule on the radius is similar to the dorsal attachment, but on the ulna, the oblique line of attachment courses in a volar direction around the neck of the ulna, almost to the ulnar styloid. This makes most of the circumference of the head of the ulna intracapsular, so the radius rotates almost 180° around the ulna.

Dorsally, the DRUJ capsule is thickened in its proximal third. Volarly, it is thickest in the distal third (Fig. 5-21). These thickenings appear to be the principal constraints to extreme pronation and supination respectively.

The ligamentum subcruetnum, about 2 mm wide, arises from the fovea of the ulna at the base of the ulnar styloid, and extends to the volar margin of the sigmoid notch of the radius. It is tight in supination but folds beneath the TFC articular disc in pronation.

The volar capsule is lax in pronation and invaginates between the radius and ulna beneath the ligamentum subcruetnum immediately proximal to the head of the ulna. The dorsal capsule is tight in pro-

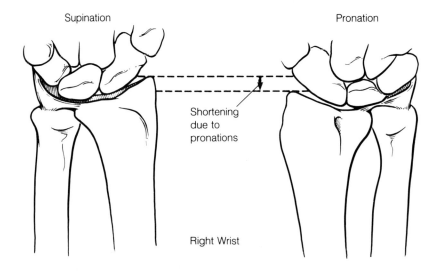

FIGURE 5–19.
Apparent radial shortening in pronation. The triangular fibrocartilage complex central disc is pulled tight over the head of the ulna and is compressed between the ulna and lunate.

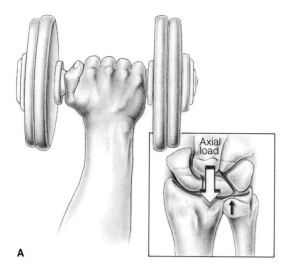

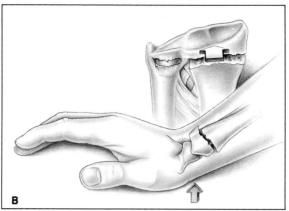

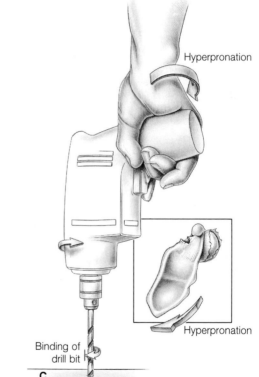

FIGURE 5–20.
Forces on the distal radioulnar joint. (**A**) Axial load. (**B**) Sagittal forces associated with radius fracture. (**C**) Rotational force caused by hyperpronation, a common injury with power tools.

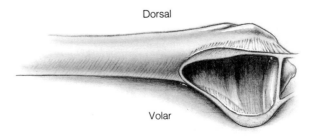

FIGURE 5–21.
The distal radioulnar joint capsule is thickened proximally in its dorsal aspect, and thickened distally in its volar aspect.

nation—especially in its thickened proximal third—and is stretched over the head of the ulna as the ulna slides dorsally. Conversely, in supination the dorsal capsule is lax as the radius rotates to approach the ulnar styloid and the volar capsule tightens, especially in its thickened distal third.

Because the radius is relatively longer in supination, it lifts the TFCC articular disc away from the ulnar head in this position. This opens the space beneath the TFCC, especially in the presence of negative ulnar variance, and facilitates arthroscopic instrumentation if the wrist is held in supination. The volar and dorsal margins of the TFCC are thickened considerably.

The anatomy of the wrist is exceedingly complex, and its intricacy is fascinating. The mechanical integration of tendons, ligaments, and articular surfaces is generally not well appreciated, but an understanding of the system is crucial to the successful evaluation of soft-tissue injuries to the wrist and to the design of appropriate treatment.

REFERENCES

1. Cooney WP, Dobyns JH, Linscheid RL. Arthroscopy of the wrist: anatomy and classification of carpal instability. Arthroscopy 1990;6(2):133.
2. Martin D, Whipple TL, Sims S, Yates C. The role of the triangular fibrocartilage complex in distal radioulnar joint stability: a cadaver study. J Hand Surg [Am] (in press).

BIBLIOGRAPHY

Belsole RJ, Hilbelink D, Llewellyn JA, Dale M, Stenzler S, Rayhack JM. The scaphoid orientation and location from computed, three dimensional carpal models. Orthop Clin North Am 1986;17(3):505.

Brumbaugh RB, Crowninshield RD, Blair WF, Andrews JG. An in vivo study of normal wrist kinematics. J Biomed Eng 1982;104(3):176.

Drewniany JJ, Palmer AK, Flatt AE. The scaphotrapezial ligament complex: an anatomic and biomechanical study. J Hand Surg [Am] 1985;10(4):492.

Fisk GR. The influence of the transverse carpal ligament (flexor retinaculum) on carpal stability. Ann Chir Main 1984;3(4):297.

Hotchkiss RN, An KN, Sowa DT, Basta S, Weiland AJ. An anatomic and mechanical study of the interosseous membrane of the forearm: pathomechanics of proximal migration of the radius. J Hand Surg [Am] 1989;14(2):256.

Kauer JM, DeLange A. The carpal joint: anatomy and function. Hand Clin 1987;3(1):23.

Kauer JM. Functional anatomy of the wrist. Clin Orthop 1980;149:9.

King GJ, McMurtry RY, Ruberstein JD, Gertzbein SD. Kinematics of the distal radioulnar joint. J Hand Surg [Am] 1986;11(6):798.

Linscheid RL. Kinematic considerations of the wrist. Clin Orthop 1986;202:27.

Logan SE, Nowak ND, Gould PL, Weeks PM. Biomechanical behavior of the scapholunate ligament. Biomed Sci Instrum 1986;22:81.

Logan SE, Nowak ND. Intrinsic and extrinsic wrist ligaments: biomechanical and functional differences. ISA Trans 1988;27(2):37.

Palmer AK. The distal radioulnar joint. Orthop Clin North Am 1984;15(2):321.

Palmer AK. The distal radioulnar joint: anatomy, biomechanics and triangular fibrocartilage complex abnormalities. Hand Clin 1987;3(1):31.

Palmer AK, Skahen JR, Werner FW, Glisson RR. The extensor retinaculum of the wrist: an anatomical and biomechanical study. J Hand Surg [Br] 1985;10(1):11.

Palmer AK, Werner FW. The triangular fibrocartilage complex of the wrist: anatomy and function. J Hand Surg [Am] 1981;6(2):153.

Ruby LK, Cooney WP III, An KN, Linscheid RL, Chao DY. Relative motion of selected carpal bones: a kinematic analysis of the normal wrist. J Hand Surg [Am] 1988;13(1):1.

Soechting JF, Terzuolo CA. An algorithm for the generation of curvilinear wrist motion in an arbitrary plane in three dimensional space. Neuroscience 1986;19(4):1393.

Sommer HJ III, Miller NR. A technique for kinematic modeling of anatomical joints. J Biomech Eng 1980;102(4):311.

Viegas SF, Tencer AF, Cantrell J, et al. Load transfer characteristics of the wrist. Part II. Perilunate instability. J Hand Surg [Am] 1987;12(6):978.

Volz RG, Lieb M, Benjamin J. Biomechanics of the wrist. Clin Orthop 1980;149:112.

Watson HK, Black DM. Instabilities of the wrist. Hand Clin 1987;3(1):103.

Youm Y, Flatt AE. Kinematics of the wrist. Clin Orthop 1980;149:21.

Zancoli EA, Ziadenberg C, Zancoli E Jr. Biomechanics of the trapeziometacarpal joint. Clin Orthop 1987;220:14.

6

Diagnostic Arthroscopic Examination

Wrist arthroscopy is a useful diagnostic modality for wrist pathology of traumatic, inflammatory, or degenerative origin. It provides a means of direct visual inspection and manipulation of the internal articular and ligamentous structures, and can be performed with little discomfort or inconvenience to the patient. Wrist arthroscopy is but one of the several means available for evaluating the wrist. It may be indicated early or secondarily in the course of assessment, depending on the nature of symptoms and preliminary findings.

There is no substitute for a thorough history of a patient's complaints. The patient history should include the duration of symptoms, frequency of occurrence, previous similar symptoms, other disorders of the same joint, and the occurrence of other coincidental joint or systemic disorders. In the case of trauma, reconstruction of the precise mechanism of injury is imperative. Familial disorders affecting the wrist are unusual but should be noted. With this background, a thorough arthroscopic examination of the wrist can be performed with specific attention to structures suspected of involvement. The diagnostic examination should include a systematic visual and manipulative evaluation of as much of the intracapsular anatomy as can be accessed.

To confirm or qualify the suspected diagnosis, begin by directing attention to the most symptomatic region. If the examination must be aborted for some reason, the most compelling information will have been obtained. Of secondary importance is a general and systematic survey of the joint to discover any associated or occult lesions that may influence treatment or prognosis of the primary disorder.

General examination begins with identification of topographical landmarks and selection of appropriate initial portals (Fig. 6-1). Table 6-1 lists the preferred portals for suspected pathology on both the radial and ulnar sides of the wrist. For examinations in which the tentative diagnosis is uncertain, portal 3-4 is recommended for the arthroscope, with the inflow placed in the 6-U or 6-R portals.[1]

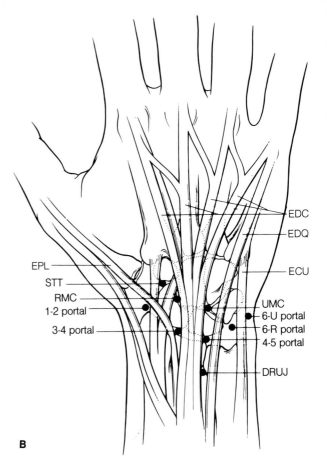

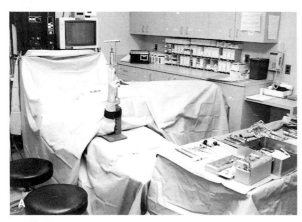

FIGURE 6—1.

(**A**) Wrist properly prepped and draped for diagnostic arthroscopic exam. Note the neat sterile field, stools for surgeon and assistant, clear view of video monitor, and access to instruments by scrub nurse, who sits facing patient's palm. (**B**) Diagram of arthroscopy portals located between extensor tendon compartments. DRUJ, distal radioulnar joint; ECU, extensor carpi ulnaris; EDC, extensor digitorum communis; EDQ, extensor digiti quinti; EPL, extensor pollicis longus; RMC, radial midcarpal portal; STT, scaphotrapeziotrapezoid; UMC, ulnar midcarpal portal.

TECHNIQUE

Using fingertraps, apply 7 to 10 pounds of traction to the index and long fingers. Mark the dorsal margin of the radius, the radial styloid, the distal end of ulna, and the ulnar styloid. Mark the proximal

Table 6—1.
PREFERRED PORTALS FOR RADIAL AND ULNAR WRIST PATHOLOGY

ARTHROSCOPE	INFLOW	ACCESSORY PORTALS
Radial Pathology		
3-4	6-U	4-5, 1-2
1-2	6-R	3-4, 4-5
Ulnar Pathology		
6-R	1-2	3-4, 6-U
6-U	1-2	4-5, 6-R

base of the second and third metacarpals. Midway between the base of the third metacarpal and the distal margin of the radius is the level of the midcarpal space. Draw the outline of extensor compartments III (extensor pollicis longus; EPL), IV (extensor digitorum communis to the index and little fingers; EDC), and VI (extensor carpi ulnaris; ECU). The ECU is a pencil-sized tendon located dorsal to the ulnar styloid.

Locate portals 3-4, 6-R, and 6-U. If accessory instruments are anticipated, locate also portals 1-2 and 4-5. Locate the radial midcarpal (RMC), ulnar midcarpal (UMC), and scaphotrapeziotrapezoid (STT) portals (see Chap. 5).

Suspected Radial Pathology

Lance the skin at 6-U and 3-4 by pulling the skin against the tip of a No. 11 scalpel. With a twisting motion introduce the inflow cannula into the 6-U

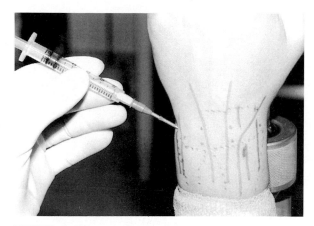

FIGURE 6–2.
Inflow cannula and syringe are oriented parallel to the proximal slope of the triquetrum before introduction through the 6-U portal. (Concept, Largo, FL.)

or the 6-R portal. The cannula should be oriented parallel to the proximal surface of triquetrum rather than parallel to the TFC, because there is less chance of piercing the TFC with this approach (Fig. 6-2). Distend the joint and connect the inflow tubing. If an infusion pump is used, connect it to the inflow cannula (Fig. 6-3). The use of a pump is completely optional. Gravity inflow is usually sufficient.

With a tapered trocar, the arthroscope sheath is introduced through the 3-4 portal. The sheath should be oriented parallel to the volar tilt of the radius (Fig. 6-4). A twisting motion is used to per-

forate the dorsal capsule. Maintain the tilted orientation of the arthroscope sheath to evacuate bubbles. Return of fluid when the trocar is removed confirms entry into the joint.

The scope enters exactly beneath the scapholunate ligament and over the sagittal ridge of the radius (Fig. 6-5). A quick visual survey of the joint is recommended because discovery of any pathology may influence the selection of portals for a probe or other accessory instruments. Usually the 4-5 portal provides the greatest instrument access to various regions of the radiocarpal space when coordinated with the arthroscope in the 3-4 portal. However, circumstances may dictate more advantageous accessory approaches from the 1-2 or 6-U portals. Placing a hypodermic needle in these portals under arthroscopic visualization will help confirm the best access to the joint.

Insertion of the Probe

After lancing the skin and spreading the subcutaneous tissue, the probe is inserted. Keeping the probe in view, examine visually and with palpation the entire articular surface of the radius. Begin with radial styloid, sagittal ridge, and the articular facets of the scaphoid and lunate (Fig. 6-6). Articular surfaces should feel smooth and slippery, with the consistency of a tomato skin.

On the volar side, note the integrity of the volar radiocarpal ligaments, beginning with the radio-

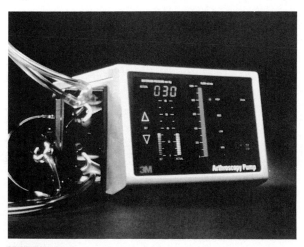

FIGURE 6–3.
Typical arthroscopy infusion pump (3-M, Minneapolis, MN). Pressure and flow rate are monitored and automatically controlled by the pump.

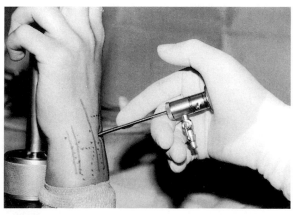

FIGURE 6–4.
Arthroscope sheath and tapered trocar are oriented parallel to the volar slope of the distal radius articular surface before entry through the 3-4 portal. Note the surgeon's finger positioned on the shaft of the arthroscope sheath to prevent an inadvertent plunge into the joint.

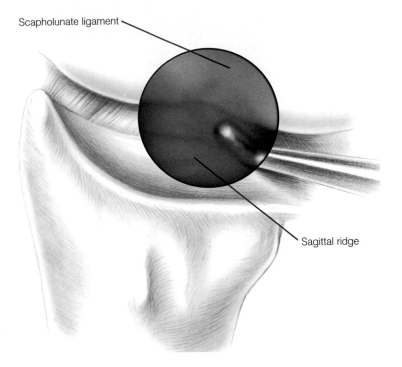

Scapholunate ligament

Sagittal ridge

FIGURE 6–5.
Initial arthroscopic view from the 3-4 portal, right wrist. Note the scapholunate ligament above, and the sagittal ridge of the radius below.

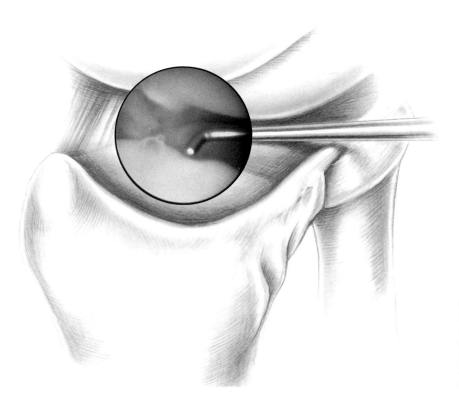

FIGURE 6–6.
Sagittal ridge of the distal radius separating the scaphoid articular facet and radial styloid from the lunate articular facet. The sagittal ridge is located immediately beneath the scapholunate ligament.

scaphocapitate (RSC), and then the radiolunotriquetral (RLT). On the volar aspect will be seen a synovial tuft adjacent to the RLT ligament and projecting into the ligament (Fig. 6-7). When retracting this structure radially with the probe, one can sometimes see the volar scapholunate ligament or ligament of Testut (Fig. 6-8). The ligament of Testut courses at a 60° to 80° angle to the slope of the RLT ligament.

Farther ulnar, the articular transition from radius to the triangular fibrocartilage complex (TFCC) may be barely discernable in the normal states. The

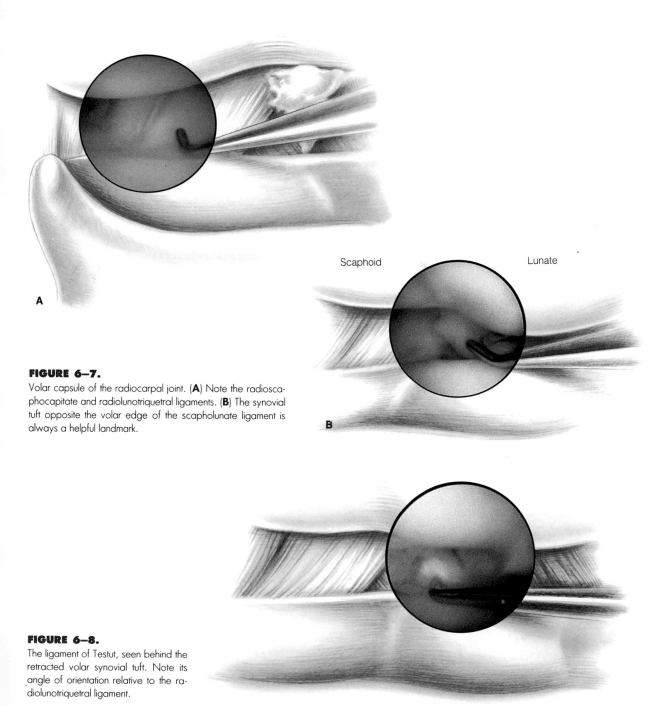

FIGURE 6–7.
Volar capsule of the radiocarpal joint. (**A**) Note the radioscaphocapitate and radiolunotriquetral ligaments. (**B**) The synovial tuft opposite the volar edge of the scapholunate ligament is always a helpful landmark.

FIGURE 6–8.
The ligament of Testut, seen behind the retracted volar synovial tuft. Note its angle of orientation relative to the radiolunotriquetral ligament.

difference can be appreciated by feeling the resistance of underlying bone on the lunate facet and the unsupported resilience of the articular disc of the TFCC (Fig. 6-9). The volar and dorsal margins of the TFCC articular disc blend smoothly with the capsule except for a 3- to 4-mm area volar to the ulnar styloid. This hiatus represents entry into the prestyloid recess (Fig. 6-10). The TFCC must be thoroughly probed to assure its integrity. The dorsal capsule here consists of the floor of the ECU tendon

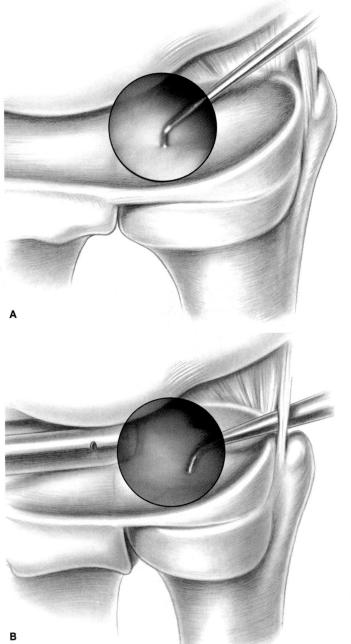

A

B

FIGURE 6–9.

The triangular fibrocartilage articular disc. (**A**) The probe has slipped just off the articular surface of the lunate facet of the radius. (**B**) The probe explores the unsupported resilience of the central portion of the disc.

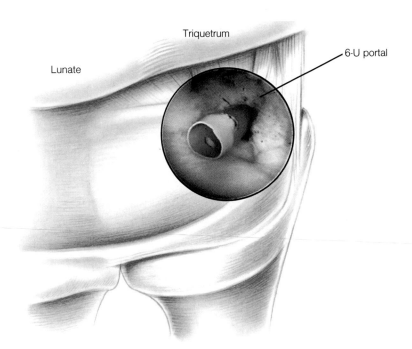

Lunate

Triquetrum

6-U portal

FIGURE 6–10.
Arthroscopic photograph (right wrist) showing inflow cannula presenting through the entrance into the prestyloid recess, a pocket in the ulnar joint capsule adjacent to the edge of the triangular fibrocartilage articular disc.

sheath. The volar capsule has longitudinal fibers representing the volar ulnocarpal ligaments. These fibers arise from the fovea of the ulna and bifurcate distally to insert on the lunate and triquetrum.

Looking distally on the ulnar side of the radiocarpal interval, the articular surface of the proximal row will be seen. The triquetrum will have a slight convex surface of articular cartilage. If the proximal row has a large radius of curvature as can be seen on the posteroanterior radiograph, the proximal pole of the triquetrum will have a relatively transverse orientation and will present a substantial articular surface in the radiocarpal space. However, if the proximal row radius of curvature is small, as in a petite wrist, the triquetrum surface will be oriented more longitudinally, and the proximal pole will have little articular cartilage (Fig. 6-11).

A slight reversal of the convex contour of the triquetrum as the scope is panned radially will mark the location of the lunotriquetral intercarpal ligament (Fig. 6-12). This is not always visible from the 3-4 portal, especially in a petite wrist with a short radius of curvature of the proximal carpal row. When palpated, the lunotriquetral ligament will feel shorter than the adjacent articular cartilage, but it will have nearly the same color as this cartilage. It

is necessary, therefore, to look for the change from a convex to a concave contour of the proximal row to identify the lunotriquetral ligament.

The articular surface of lunate is again convex and feels firm and slippery. In a neutral wrist position, approximately one-half of the lunate will articulate with the TFC and the other one-half will articulate with the lunate facet of the radius. At the radial edge of the lunate, the proximal row contour again becomes concave, showing the location of the scapholunate ligament. The scapholunate ligament is wider than the lunotriquetral ligament. The color and texture may be very similar to the articular cartilage, but with age the ligament becomes fibrillated and slightly more yellow than the adjacent cartilage of the lunate and scaphoid (Fig. 6-13).

At the most volar edge of the scapholunate ligament is the synovial tuft, which projects into the radiocarpal space from the volar capsule (see Fig. 6-7B). This is an important landmark for visual orientation. From this structure one can easily locate the volar radiocarpal ligament, the sagittal ridge of the radius, the scapholunate ligament, and the articular surfaces of the lunate and scaphoid.

The proximal articular surface of the scaphoid resembles that of the lunate. On examining these

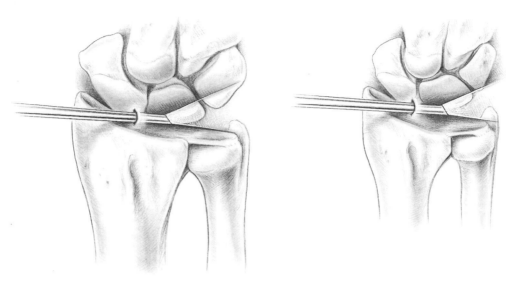

FIGURE 6–11.
Arthroscopic view of the proximal articular surface of the triquetrum in large and petite wrists. Note the more vertical orientation of the triquetrum in the petite specimen, and the inability to see this surface arthroscopically from the 3-4 portal. The triquetrum is more readily visible from the 3-4 portal in larger patients, who have a more transverse orientation of the proximal carpal row.

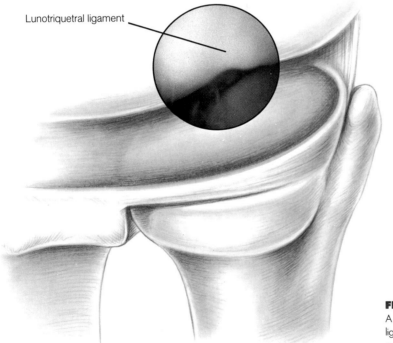

Lunotriquetral ligament

FIGURE 6–12.
A slight concave contour represents the lunotriquetral ligament between the convex contours of the triquetrum and the lunate.

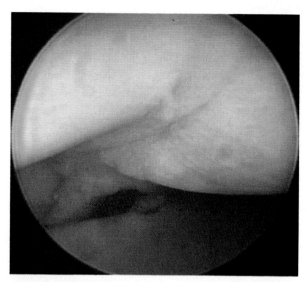

FIGURE 6—13.
Scapholunate ligament in a 64-year-old patient (right wrist). Note the slight fibrillation, folding, and yellowish discoloration of the ligament.

hypertrophy to villi, ranging in color from white to salmon pink to red (Fig. 6-16).

Suspected Ulnar Pathology

More extensive examination of the ulnar side of the radiocarpal interval may be required if ulnar pathology is strongly suspected. In these circumstances, the arthroscope should be introduced in the 6-R portal after establishing an inflow cannula in the 1-2 portal. This will position the inflow system out of the way if other operative instruments are needed on the ulnar side. The 3-4 or 6-U portals may be advantageous for accessory instruments on the ulnar side of the radiocarpal space.

From the 6-R portal a good view of the TFCC can be obtained, except for where it merges with the dorsal capsule. The attachment of the ulnar capsule to the triquetrum is visible. On the volar capsule, the ulnocarpal ligament can be seen bifurcating into two distinct bundles distally to insert on the lunate and triquetrum (Fig. 6-17). This bifurcation is usually not visible from the 3-4 portal. The articular surface of the triquetrum and lunotriquetral ligament can also be better seen from the 6-R portal.

Usually the pisotriquetral joint will communicate with the radiocarpal space. This may occur through the prestyloid recess, or there may be a separate aperture located volar and distal to the prestyloid recess (Fig. 6-18). It is often possible to advance

surfaces, the wrist should be gently flexed and extended to reveal essentially all of the volar and dorsal portions of the cartilage (Fig. 6-14).

More radially, the joint capsule arches to attach to the scaphoid. The normal synovial lining of the joint capsule is smooth and thin (Fig. 6-15). If inflamed, a lacy pattern of small capillaries can be seen. In chronic inflammatory states, the synovium will

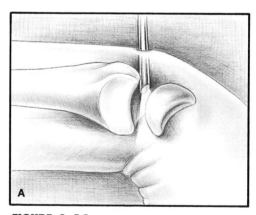
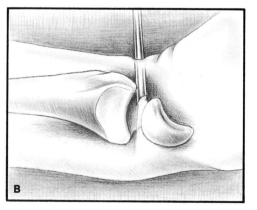

FIGURE 6—14.
(**A**) Flexion and (**B**) extension of the wrist provide greater visual access to the dorsal and volar articular surfaces of the lunate and the proximal pole of the scaphoid.

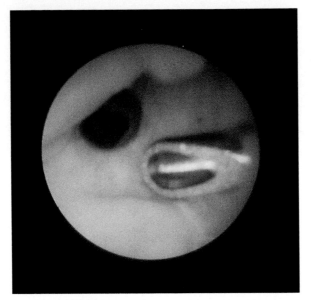

FIGURE 6—15.
Normal synovial lining of the ulnar joint capsule (right wrist). Note the low-profile, smooth, white appearance of the synovium.

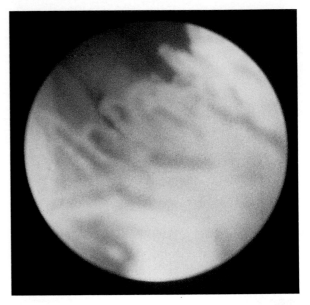

FIGURE 6—16.
Inflamed hypertrophic synovium in the ulnar joint capsule. Note the elongated, edematous villi with varying color and engorged capillaries.

a 1.9-mm arthroscope into these capsular openings and see the ulnar edge of the pisotriquetral articulation (Fig. 6-19). From the 6-R portal, one will be looking toward the articular surface of pisiform. Loose bodies have been found in both the pisotriquetral space and in the prestyloid recess.

Other Vantage Points

Finally, there are occasional circumstances when obtaining a view of certain parts of the radiocarpal space requires placement of the arthroscope in one of the portals usually used for accessory instruments. The dorsal capsule and its attachments to the proximal row are seen best from the vantage of the 1-2 portal. When looking for intraarticular ganglia or avulsion injuries to the dorsal capsule, it is advisable to use this approach (Fig. 6-20). The arthroscope may be the largest instrument to be placed in the 1-2 portal. Extreme care should be taken to avoid injury to the radial artery. To do so, the portals should be established in the 1-2 interval immediately adjacent to the intersection of the extensor carpi radialis longus (ECRL) and the EPL. The radial artery is located in the volar aspect of the anatomic snuffbox. Placing the 1-2 portal as dorsal as possible and

spreading the subcutaneous tissue with a hemostat down to the level of the joint capsule is the most reliable means of protecting this important vessel.

Injury to the volar ulnar aspect of the wrist that involves the ulnocarpal ligaments or fractures of the

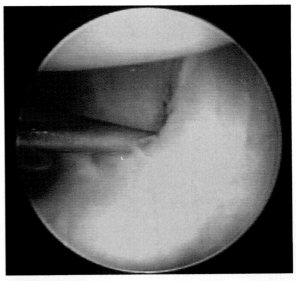

FIGURE 6—17.
Bifurcation of the volar ulnocarpal ligaments as seen from the 6-R portal. On the left is the ulnolunate ligament. On the right is the ulnotriquetral ligament. The probe approaches from the 3-4 portal.

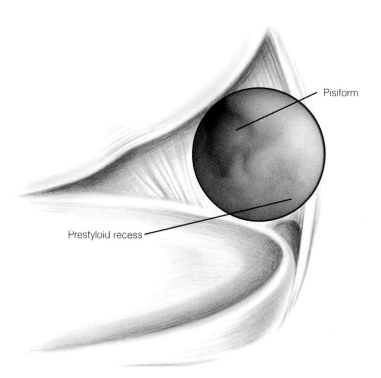

Pisiform

Prestyloid recess

FIGURE 6–18.
A separate opening of the ulnar joint capsule into the pisotriquetral joint appears at the ulnar margin of the ulnotriquetral ligament.

triquetrum may require examination through the 6-U portal. This is the only approach from which the most distal portion of the ulnocarpal ligaments can be examined. The arthroscope will enter the joint through the prestyloid recess. When the wrist is flexed, the volar attachments of the capsule and ligaments to the proximal carpal row can be seen (Fig. 6-21).

Examination of the Midcarpal Space

The midcarpal space of the wrist is easier to access than might be imagined. Although pathology is encountered here less frequently than in the radiocarpal space, much information can be gleaned from arthroscopic examination of this interval. The RMC portal is invariably used for the arthroscope.

Lance the skin by drawing it against the tip of a No. 11 scalpel as described previously. Introduce the arthroscope sheath with a blunt trocar into the midcarpal space between the scaphoid and capitate, using a twisting motion to perforate the dorsal capsule. As there is no normal communication between the radiocarpal space and the midcarpal space, inflow fluid is delivered through the arthroscope sheath (Fig. 6-22).

To avoid the introduction of air bubbles into the joint, the sheath must be pointed in a proximal direction. Open the inflow line, and connect it to the sheath before slowly withdrawing the trocar. The sheath will fill with fluid, displacing bubbles toward

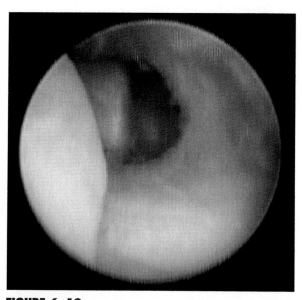

FIGURE 6–19.
The pisotriquetral articulation (right wrist) as seen from the 6-R portal with a 1.9-mm arthroscope.

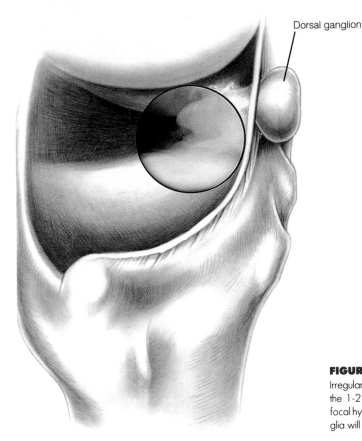

Dorsal ganglion

FIGURE 6—20.

Irregular synovium around the stoma of a dorsal ganglion seen from the 1-2 portal (right wrist). The opening itself is rarely visible, but the focal hypertrophic synovium is almost always present. Intraarticular ganglia will appear as single cysts or small clusters of cysts in this location.

the extraarticular end of the sheath. Tap the sheath to dislodge any additional bubbles, then insert the arthroscope. The midcarpal space should be examined systematically, looking first for pathology that may be suspected.

Through the RMC portal, the arthroscope enters the midcarpal space between the scaphoid and the capitate. The concave articular surface of the scaphoid is almost always smooth and intact (Fig. 6-23). Rarely is any abnormality encountered here unless the scaphoid has been fractured. Follow the scaphoid contour distally to the STT interval. The articular surface of the distal pole of the scaphoid will be oriented transversely. Looking distally, the trapezium and trapezoid can be seen; the trapezium will be in the background, the trapezoid in the foreground (Fig. 6-24). Degenerative changes are common in the STT articulation. Their severity may be assessed by probing the surfaces with a probe through the STT portal. It is not unusual to find

the distal pole of scaphoid completely devoid of hyaline cartilage.

Any bubbles introduced inadvertently in the midcarpal space will usually collect at the STT interval with the forearm suspended vertically. Evacuate them to clear the visual field by inserting a hypodermic needle through the STT portal. The positive inflow pressure will force the bubbles out when they are touched with the needle.

As the scope is passed back along the concave surface of the scaphoid, the scapholunate interval will present proximally. There are no intrinsic intercarpal ligaments in the midcarpal space, so this interval can be easily recognized. Marginal fraying of the articular cartilage along the scapholunate interval when the remainder of the surface appears normal may indicate rotatory subluxation of the scaphoid (Fig. 6-25). This is a subtle but significant sign.

There may be one or two articular facets on the

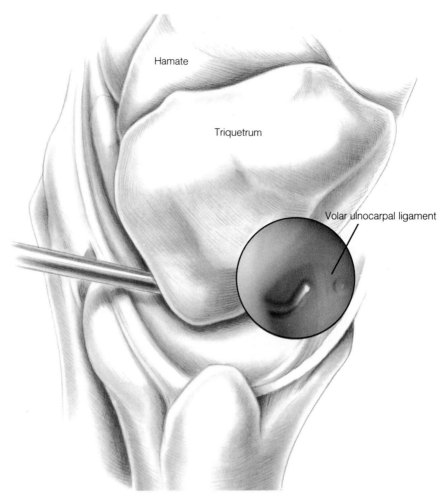

Hamate

Triquetrum

Volar ulnocarpal ligament

FIGURE 6–21.
Volar attachment of the joint capsule to the proximal row seen from the 6-U portal (right wrist). The probe enters from the 4-5 portal and passes beneath the lunotriquetral ligament.

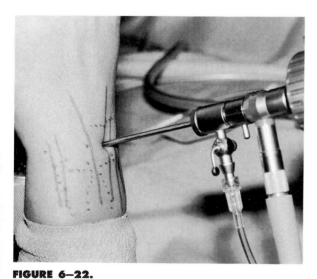

FIGURE 6–22.
The arthroscope in the radial midcarpal portal (left wrist). Note the connection of the inflow line to the arthroscope sheath.

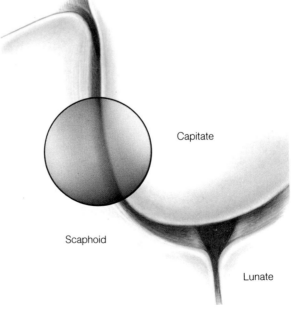

Capitate

Scaphoid

Lunate

FIGURE 6–23.
The first view of the smooth scaphocapitate articulation on entering the midcarpal space through the radial midcarpal portal (right wrist).

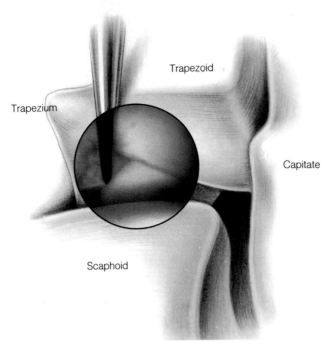

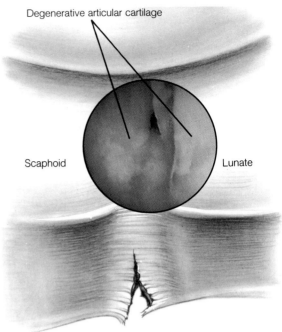

FIGURE 6–24.
The scaphotrapeziotrapezoid (STT) joint seen through the radial midcarpal portal (right wrist). The needle enters through the STT portal and points to the trapezium in the background. Normally, there is no intrinsic ligament visible between the trapezium and trapezoid.

FIGURE 6–25.
Degenerative changes in the articular cartilage along the margins of the scaphoid and lunate in the midcarpal space seen through the radial midcarpal portal (right wrist). This condition is frequently observed in dynamic scapholunate dissociation, even without disruption of the scaphoid ligament.

distal surface of lunate (Fig. 6-26). One accommodates the head of the capitate; a smaller one may exist for the proximal pole of the hamate but is an inconsistent finding on the lunate.[2]

The lunotriquetral interval should be examined for symmetry. The gap is normally the same width anterior to posterior. The triquetrum can be manipulated by dorsal and volar pressure while examining the lunotriquetral interval. Although the triquetrum may rock relative to the lunate, there normally should be no anterior to posterior translation movement between the carpal bones. Examine the saddle-shaped joint of the hamate and triquetrum. The articulation between these two bones should be held very tight by the volar triquetro-hamate-capitate (THC) ligament. If this interval can be widely distracted by traction or radial deviation so that the volar ligament can be seen well, midcarpal instability (MCI) is likely present (Fig. 6-27). Another sign of MCI is an articular defect on the extreme proximal

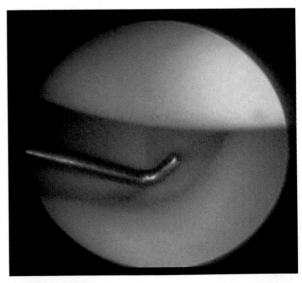

FIGURE 6–26.
Two distinct distal articular facets are seen on the lunate from the radial midcarpal portal (right wrist). The facets accommodate the capitate and hamate respectively.

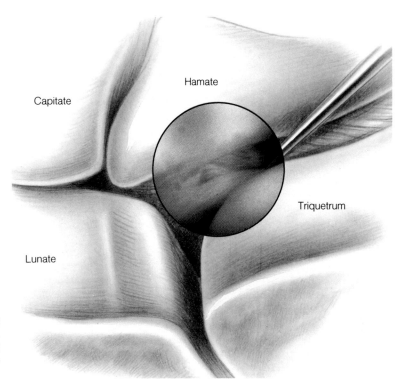

FIGURE 6–27.

A distracted, saddle-shaped triquetrohamate joint (right wrist). The lax, edematous fibers of the triquetrohamate ligament are associated with midcarpal instability. The probe is inserted through the ulnar midcarpal portal.

pole of the hamate (Fig 6-28). This lesion may exist for other reasons as well, but in MCI it is presumed to be caused by the forceful articulation of hamate against the ulnar edge of lunate in ulnar deviation of the wrist. As the lunate then shifts from a volar intercalated segmental instability (VISI) to a dorsal intercalated segmental instability (DISI) orientation, the shearing motion damages the hamate.

The ulnar capsule of the midcarpal space should be examined. Finally, look for articular changes on the head of the capitate. If a probe or other accessory operating instrument is required on the ulnar side of the midcarpal space, the UMC portal is convenient and can be entered with ease at the articular junction of the lunate, triquetrum, hamate, and capitate (Fig. 6-29).

Distal Radioulnar Joint

Arthroscopic examination of the distal radioulnar joint (DRUJ) can be difficult and is not always pos-

sible. The interosseous membrane, among other structures, holds the ulna closely applied to the sigmoid notch of the radius. Without DRUJ instability, this joint cannot be distracted. However, when the forearm is supinated, the head of the ulna shifts in a volar direction and the dorsal capsule of the DRUJ becomes lax (Fig. 5-6C). In this position, the joint can be distended with a hypodermic needle, and the arthroscope may be introduced dorsally between the fourth and fifth extensor compartments proximal to the sigmoid notch of the radius. Here a sharp trocar is recommended because the arthroscope does not directly approach articular cartilage. The capsule can be seen, as can the metaphysis of the distal ulna (Fig. 6-30). Loose bodies are occasionally encountered in this proximal aspect of the distal radioulnar joint. Synovitis may be prevalent in inflammatory arthritides.

The dorsal aspect of the sigmoid notch may be visible, but never the volar aspect, unless the DRUJ is extremely unstable. If the scope is held stationary in a position relative to the radius, slow pronation

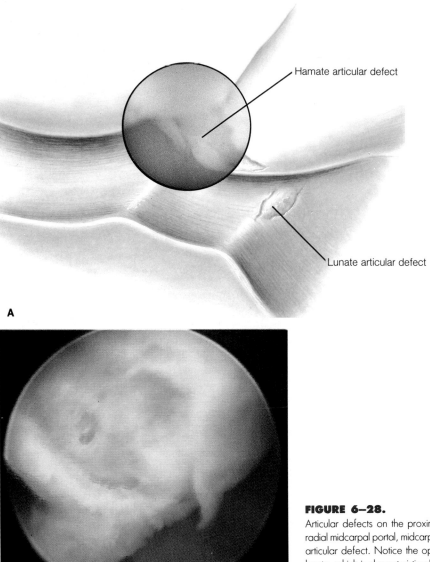

Hamate articular defect

Lunate articular defect

A

B

FIGURE 6–28.

Articular defects on the proximal pole of the hamate seen through the radial midcarpal portal, midcarpal space (right wrist). (**A**) A minor superficial articular defect. Notice the opposing defect on the ulnar margin of the lunate, which is characteristic of midcarpal instability. (**B**) Notice the frayed edge of cartilage (*right*), the vertical shoulder of hyaline (*lower left*), and the roughened subchondral bone.

of the forearm will parade the articular surface of the ulna in front of the arthroscope for a limited view. If negative ulnar variance is present, a more proximal introduction of the arthroscope into the DRUJ may be possible. Again, the forearm is placed in supination (anatomic position) to maintain maximal length of the radius relative to the ulna. After distending the joint with a hypodermic needle, a

blunt trocar is used to introduce the arthroscope sheath immediately proximal and ulnar to the palpable distal ulnar corner of the radius. The scope will enter the joint between tendons of the EDC, proximal to the TFCC attachment to the radius. This space is small, but it is still sometimes possible to see the proximal surface of TFCC articular disc and the cartilage-covered head of the distal ulna (Fig.

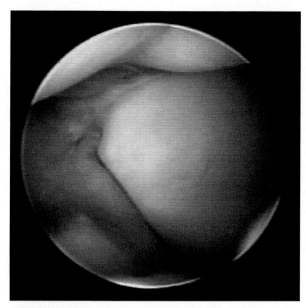

FIGURE 6—29.
The midcarpal space seen through the ulnar midcarpal portal (right wrist). The first view is that of the intersecting articulations between the capitate and hamate above, and the lunate and triquetrum below.

6-31). The value of this approach to the DRUJ is uncertain, however, and multiple attempts at entry are not recommended, since the TFCC or DRUJ may be injured in the effort.

POSTOPERATIVE MANAGEMENT

Discomfort following diagnostic arthroscopy of the wrist is not great, and it does not take long for the portals to heal. Sutures are unnecessary for the 2- to 3-mm punctures. A sterile compressive bandage is applied from the metacarpophalangeal joints to the midforearm, incorporating a volar plaster splint if partial immobilization is desired (Fig. 6-32). Elevation for 24 hours is recommended to deter bleeding from dorsal veins that may have been injured. The Ringer's solution that has extravasated into subcutaneous tissues is usually absorbed in a few hours. The bandage can be removed in 3 to 5 days, and if the skin punctures are sealed, bathing may be

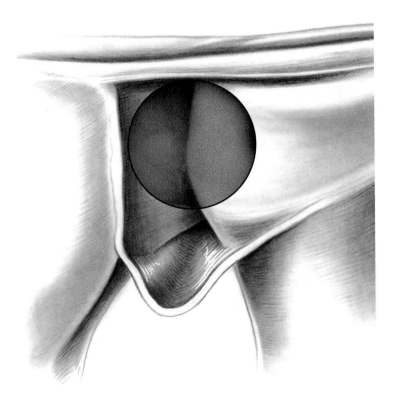

FIGURE 6—30.
The distal radioulnar joint (right wrist). Note the convex contour of the ulnar head, and the concave contour of the sigmoid notch of the radius.

Volar ulnocarpal ligaments

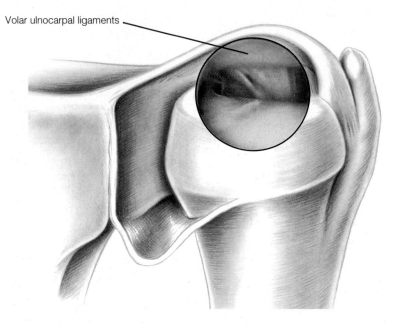

FIGURE 6–31.
A view of the proximal surface of the triangular fibrocartilage articular disc in the distal radioulnar joint. Note the origin of the ulnotriquetral ligament in the background.

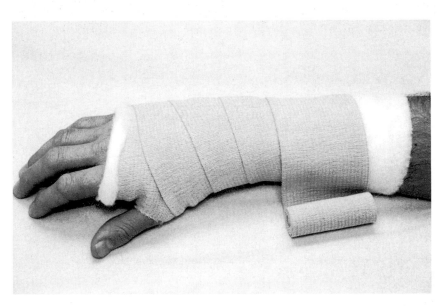

FIGURE 6–32.
Postoperative dressing consists of a padded compression bandage. A volar plaster splint may be incorporated.

permitted. Should a portal remain moist, however, painting the skin frequently with an antiseptic solution will help to reduce the risk of contamination of the superficial joint. Resumption of functional activity depends on the diagnosis but need not be otherwise delayed because of the arthroscopic examination.

BIBLIOGRAPHY

Whipple TL, Marotta JJ, Powell JH III. Techniques of wrist arthroscopy. Arthroscopy 1986;2(4):244.

Viegas SF. Intraarticular ganglion of the dorsal interosseous scapholunate ligament: a case for arthroscopy. Arthroscopy 1986;2(2):93.

Section Two

Surgical Arthroscopy

7

Articular Surface Defects and Loose Bodies

*C*arpal bones develop from ossification of cartilage anlage (Fig. 7-1). The carpal cartilage shell is therefore thick and soft before skeletal maturity and progressively ossifies with age, becoming thinner and more firm.

As the wrist sustains impact and shearing loads, insidious wear and articular trauma are inevitable. Defects on the normally smooth and slippery articular surface are far more common than might be expected. Poehling and colleagues observed articular lesions in 64% of wrists consecutively examined by arthroscopy.[1] Subluxation associated with carpal instability subjects the articular surfaces of the wrist to unusual shearing forces, and can produce abnormal premature wear patterns over time. Acute trauma such as carpal dislocation or intraarticular fracture not only causes the obvious ligament and bone injuries seen in radiographs, but damages articular surfaces as well.

Although the wrist is not as much a load-bearing joint as the ankle or knee, articular defects in the wrist do progress in size and depth, even with normal use. Slight to moderate defects may cause troublesome symptoms, but they are usually not recognizable with routine or even sophisticated imaging techniques. Arthroscopic examination will identify articular defects more consistently than any other diagnostic measure (Fig. 7-2).

Many articular lesions are untreatable. However, knowing their presence, location, and severity will explain certain symptoms and indicate appropriate precautions for limiting or modifying activity. Arthroscopy provides the opportunity to palpate the even, smooth articular surfaces to identify areas of softening or detachment of cartilage from subchondral bone (Fig. 7-3).

Abrasion, fracture, or other sloughing of articular cartilage can produce loose bodies in the wrist joint. If these fragments are small, they are invested by synovial villi and absorbed by enzymatic degradation. Proteolytic enzymes are produced by the surface intimal cells of the synovial membrane. Release of these enzymes into joint fluid has the same digestive effect on intact hyaline cartilage as on free fragments. This chemical insult to normal cartilage can be blocked by the use of antiinflammatory medications, but at the expense of impeding the cleansing function of the synovium.

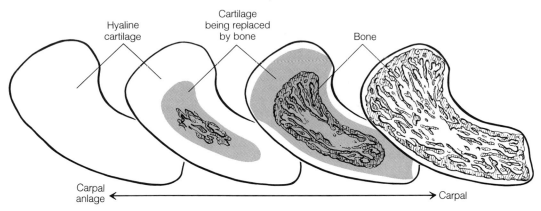

Hyaline cartilage

Cartilage being replaced by bone

Bone

Carpal anlage

Carpal

FIGURE 7–1.
Progressive ossification of a carpal anlage with age. Note that the articular surface becomes thinner and more firm because of the expanding bone within.

Joint debris can also be removed from the wrist by arthroscopic lavage or arthroscopic surgery. In severely degenerated joints, the procedure may need to be repeated periodically. Mechanical cleansing of the joint keeps the inflammatory process in check and helps to preserve remaining articular surfaces.

Common sources of articular defects and loose bodies include direct or repetitive trauma, intraarticular fractures, cartilage nutritional disorders, and infection. Liberal use of intraarticular steroids by injection can also break down cartilage. The most common cause is simple chronic wear with aging (Fig. 7-4). The rate of wear may be influenced by genetic factors, which determine among other things the durability of the collagen helixes and fibrillar matrix. Although all articular surfaces are susceptible to wear, there appear to be common patterns to degenerative change.

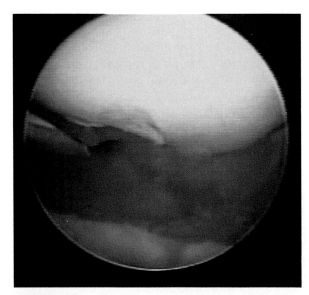

FIGURE 7–2.
Outerbridge grade III articular defect on the proximal pole of the lunate (right wrist).

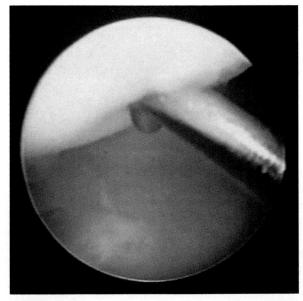

FIGURE 7–3.
Localized articular softening (Outerbridge, grade I) on the proximal lunate (right wrist).

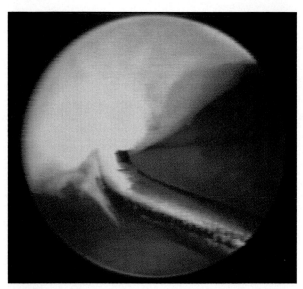

CHAPTER 7

FIGURE 7–4.
Superficial fraying of lamina splendins secondary to sheer stress on the proximal pole of the scaphoid (right wrist). The probe enters through the 4-5 portal.

Compression and shearing forces are significant stresses. Hyaline cartilage in all joints appears to withstand loads of 20 kg/cm^2. These are simple loads, however, and it is not well understood how effectively shearing forces under load are tolerated.

Wrist joint surfaces that frequently show signs of wear include the carpometacarpal (CMC) joint of the thumb, the distal pole of the scaphoid, and the radioscaphoid articulation. Less commonly affected are the head of the capitate, the proximal pole of the hamate, and the acetabular surfaces of the scaphoid and lunate that cradle the capitate. Only late in age is the radiolunate articulation significantly worn down, except in cases of specific traumatic insult. The distal radioulnar joint (DRUJ) sees considerable shear through pronation and supination, but relatively little load. This articulation rarely wears appreciably except in the case of trauma or congenital deformity of the forearm.

Other articular surfaces in the wrist are relatively spared from degenerative wear. It is especially unusual to see articular wear between bones in the same carpal row. This phenomenon might be explained by the same reasons noted for DRUJ. An exception is the articular degeneration between the trapezium and trapezoid, but the ulnar osteophytes commonly seen on the trapezium articulate more with the second metacarpal than with the trapezoid.

The presence of intrinsic ligament injury and associated carpal instability alter normal load and shear patterns. Unconventional wear patterns may be seen in such circumstances. Watson has thoroughly described the typical pattern of articular degeneration occurring in scapholunate advanced collapse (SLAC) wrist.[2] The earliest changes develop at the radioscaphoid articulation and progress to the capitolunate articulation. Radiolunate surfaces are generally spared in this condition. Intraarticular fractures produce more joint debris than is generally appreciated. Attention is naturally focused on the bone, but cartilage shards and bone crumbs may be sprayed into the joint and cannot be seen on routine radiographs or even on tomograms, computed tomography scans, or magnetic resonance images. Arthroscopic examination reveals these fragments readily. They can usually be washed, picked, or shaved from the joint, leaving surfaces much more clean and less abrasive.

CLINICAL PRESENTATION

Symptoms from articular defects in the wrist are comparatively less severe or better tolerated than in the lower extremities because the wrist is a non–weight-bearing joint and motion is more easily splinted voluntarily. Patients with articular defects of traumatic origin usually present in acute stages with complaints related to some more compelling associated injury. Ligament injuries or possibly an adjacent fracture may be present. Treated with splinting or appropriate fracture care, these associated injuries resolve in days to weeks, but the articular defects do not heal. They linger, causing pain when directly loaded or firmly palpated. If questioned carefully, patients can usually identify a specific region of the wrist and certain positions that are most bothersome.

If a site is identified as locally tender and there are no other outward signs of inflammation, an articular defect should be suspected. The absence of pain on traction helps to differentiate articular lesions from local ligament injuries and heightens this suspicion. Of less differential value is reproduction of pain at extremes of passive motion, because this not only compresses articular surfaces but places tension on specific ligaments that may be injured concurrently. Degenerative articular defects may also produce localized areas of tenderness over bony prominences. However, these patients usually complain primarily of generalized aching with occasional radiation proximally or distally. There is often a history of stiffness after periods of rest and improved function after a few minutes of activity.

Radiographs are normal for traumatic articular lesions unless the underlying bone is fractured. In longstanding degenerative lesions, the joint spaces will appear narrowed, and osseous contours will be sclerotic with sharper corners or osteophyte formation. Bone scans should be positive in either event, more focal in the traumatic articular lesions. Other imaging studies are of no value for assessing articular defects.

Symptoms of localized pain—especially with motion under loaded conditions—when radiographs, arthrography, and ligament testing are normal should raise suspicion of an articular cartilage defect or loose body in the joint. Arthroscopy is indicated if symptoms are severe enough to warrant treatment or if the circumstances of a particular injury demand a confirmed diagnosis. Personal injury

and workers' compensation cases may compel a diagnosis by arthroscopic examination even when treatment might be unlikely.

ARTHROSCOPIC APPEARANCE

It is usually possible to appreciate some signs of acute chondral defects on arthroscopic examination. Edges of the lesion appear sharp or undermined, but without general fibrillation. Traumatic articular lesions are found most commonly on the scaphoid facet of the radius or the proximal pole of the scaphoid, on the head of the capitate, and on the proximal pole of the hamate (Fig. 7-5). Degenerative lesions are most prevalent in the scaphotrapeziotrapezoid (STT) articulation on the sagittal ridge of the radius, but then follow the same general distribution pattern as traumatic lesions (Fig. 7-6). Although articular defects may occur anywhere in the wrist, these common locations reflect either loading patterns or shear concentration in the wrist. Notably, the triquetrum and radiolunate articular surfaces are relatively spared. Chronic lesions will show a greater degree of fuzzy fibrillation on the surface and the edges of

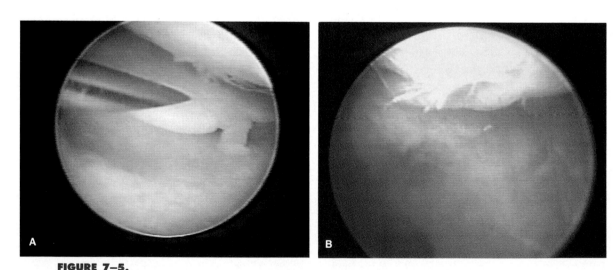

FIGURE 7–5.
(**A**) Full-thickness articular defect on the scaphoid facet of the radius. Note the undermined flap of loose articular cartilage (right wrist). (**B**) Degenerative articular changes on the head of the capitate secondary to scapholunate advanced collapse wrist.

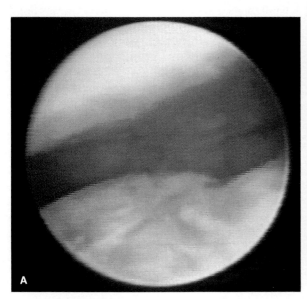

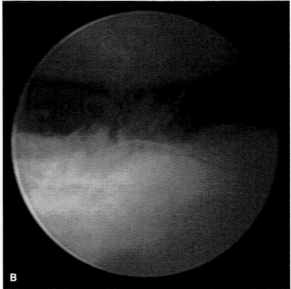

FIGURE 7–6.

(**A**) A degenerative articular defect on the distal pole of the scaphoid in the scaphotrapeziotrapezoid joint (right wrist). (**B**) Degenerative articular changes on the sagittal ridge of the radius, as viewed through the 1-2 portal (right wrist).

the defect, and may be tan or yellow (Fig. 7-7). Synovial hypertrophy may have a similar appearance in association with either acute or chronic articular

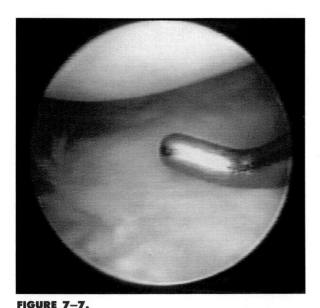

FIGURE 7–7.

A degenerative articular defect with cobblestone appearance on the scaphoid facet of the radial styloid (right wrist).

defects, but in acute synovitis the villi may be more waxy or shiny than in chronic lesions.

TREATMENT

Limited experience has been gathered from attempts to treat specific articular defects in the wrist. Fusion, joint replacement, and arthroscopic shaving are the usual approaches. The goal of arthroscopic shaving is simply to reduce the friction between opposing irregular surfaces during motion, or to obviate the natural, inflammatory, enzymatic response that follows particle sloughing. There has been no confirmed evidence of hyaline cartilage healing or regeneration after a simple shaving or debridement. If shaving or debridement is accomplished through a conventional arthrotomy, it would necessitate detachment of certain capsular ligaments to access major portions of the articular surface. This in turn can render the wrist more unstable, but usually results in stiffness from capsular scarring; hence the appeal of the arthroscopic approach.

Focal articular lesions may be caused by impact loading, acute carpal dislocation or chondral fractures associated with an acute ligamentous injury. Treatment of localized lesions by abrasion or drilling under arthroscopic control has theoretical appeal. If a blood clot can be formed in a localized articular defect, gentle motion can transform that clot into a fibrocartilage patch to fill the defect. This procedure has proved experimentally successful in a rabbit model by Salter,[3] and has been variably successful clinically in load-bearing joints such as the knee and ankle.[4] The fibrocartilage patch will bond firmly to intact adjacent hyaline cartilage. Its durability is uncertain, but by filling the articular defect it seems to offer protection against enlargement of the lesion. If the procedure is successful in certain well-circumscribed defects on load-bearing surfaces, it may be even more suitable for the wrist. Debridement and abrasion of a full-thickness Outerbridge grade IV articular defect can be accomplished arthroscopically, exposing subchondral vascular elements to produce the desired clot (Figs. 7-8 through 7-13).

I have had limited experience with this procedure in the wrist. For lesions less than 5 mm in diameter, however, symptoms have been subjectively improved without loss of wrist motion. The procedure is probably not suitable for global or even localized osteoarthritis. These conditions produce articular defects without thick adjacent shoulders of hyaline cartilage to contain a blood clot. However, small focal lesions on articular surfaces that extend deep into the hyaline cartilage appear to be reasonable indications for abrasion arthroplasty as a palliative if not a curative measure.

Chronically exposed subchondral bone on articular surfaces is a dilemma. Full-thickness degenerative lesions with bone eburnation are probably best left alone after debridement and lavage of the joint. Fusion or joint replacement offer salvage options when symptoms are severe, but many patients can achieve symptomatic relief for months with debridement and copious lavage alone.

Arthroscopic access to most of the articular surfaces in the wrist can be gained through coordinated portals in the radiocarpal and midcarpal spaces with relatively little surgical trauma. Proximally, the 3-4 and 1-2 combination or the 6-R and 3-4 combination are most useful. In the midcarpal space, the scope in the radial midcarpal (RMC) portal is combined with accessory instruments in the STT or the ulnar midcarpal (UMC) portals, depending on the location of the articular lesions.

Power shavers are an effective means of remov-

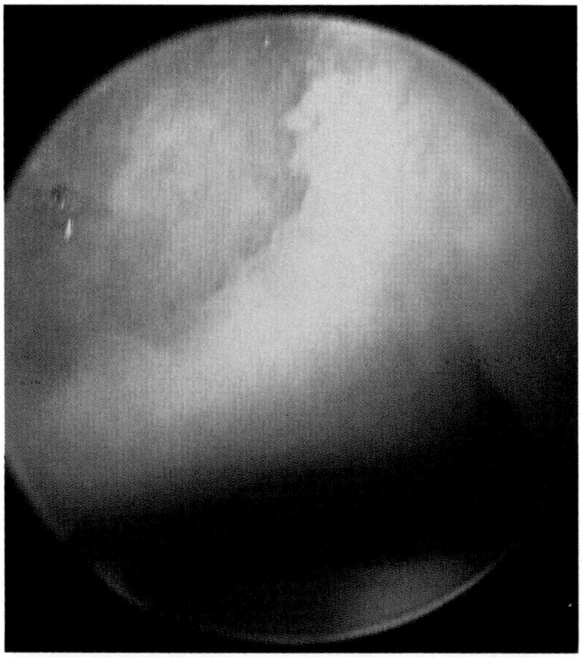

FIGURE 7-8.
A full-thickness articular defect on the proximal pole of the scaphoid, as viewed from the 1-2 portal. Vertical shoulders of hyaline cartilage surrounding this focal lesion have been shaped with a cupped curette (right wrist).

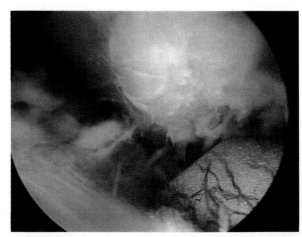

FIGURE 7-9.
A high-speed abrader preparing to debride an irregular full-thickness articular defect on the proximal pole of the scaphoid, as viewed from the 3-4 portal with burr in the 4-5 portal (right wrist).

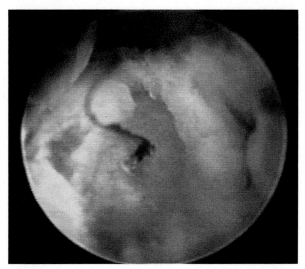

FIGURE 7–10.
Exposed vascular elements following abrasion of a full-thickness articular defect (Outerbridge, grade IV).

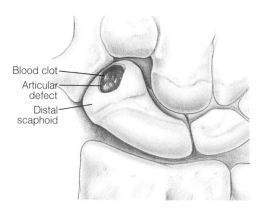

FIGURE 7–11.
An organized blood clot filling in an articular defect in the distal pole of the scaphoid after abrasion. The clot is contained and stabilized by the vertical shoulders of hyaline cartilage surrounding the defect.

ing filiform strands of degenerative hyaline cartilage (Fig. 7-14). Shavers are also most effective for smoothing the edges of ulcerated defects in hyaline cartilage. Thicker flaps of cartilage are more easily debrided with a suction punch or blunt basket

forceps that allows cutting very close to the bone (Fig. 7-15).

PREFERRED TREATMENT

It is best to approach the loose bodies identified on radiographs before any other procedures are performed. Confirm the location of the loose body preoperatively by repeating radiographs on the day of surgery. Select an arthroscope portal located closest to the loose body, whether the fragment is located in the central portion of the joint or in the periphery.

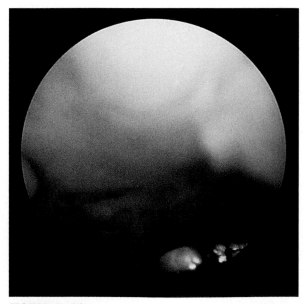

FIGURE 7–12.
Transformation of an organized blood clot into a fibrocartilage patch in full-thickness articular defect of the proximal pole of scaphoid 6 weeks after abrasion (right wrist).

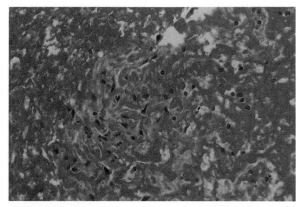

FIGURE 7–13.
Fibrous cellular differentiation within an organized clot 16 weeks after abrasion arthroplasty on the right triquetrum. Note the spindle cells in the amorphous collagen matrix. (H & E stain; original magnification ×200.)

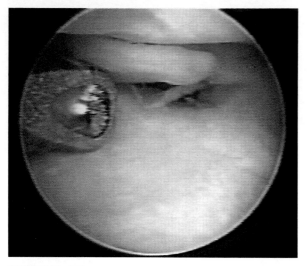

FIGURE 7–14.
A power shaver removes strands of degenerative hyaline cartilage on the proximal pole of the scaphoid and the scaphoid facet of the radius. The larger cartilage fragment will be morselized and removed with a suction punch.

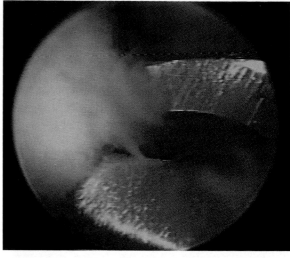

FIGURE 7–15.
A blunt basket forceps used for removing thicker flaps of articular cartilage. The blunt lower jaw facilitates cartilage resection very close to the underlying bone.

Inflow should be established away from the loose body location if possible. Suction placed on the arthroscope sheath will help to deliver loose bodies into the visual field. Access to the fragment is then achieved with a 21-gauge hypodermic needle to identify portal placement for a grasping forceps. If a safe conventional portal placement cannot be established to access the loose fragment, the hypodermic needle is used to maneuver the fragment to a position where it can be reached by a grasping forceps. Alternatively, the fragment can be speared with a hypodermic needle to immobilize it while a small arthrotomy is made to remove it.

Radiolucent loose bodies are removed in the same manner. If the fragment is large and cannot be removed intact, it should be immobilized with the needle and morselized with a suction punch or a powered shaver. Fibrillated articular surfaces are shaved only to remove loose tags of cartilage, taking care never to deepen the defect. Even fibrillated cartilage is considered better than an exposed, smooth, subchondral bone surface. Isolated full-thickness defects resulting from trauma are contoured with a cup or ring curette to create vertical shoulders of stable hyaline cartilage around the lesion. A 2- to 3-mm power burr or a strong curette is then used to abrade the subchondral bone without tourniquet

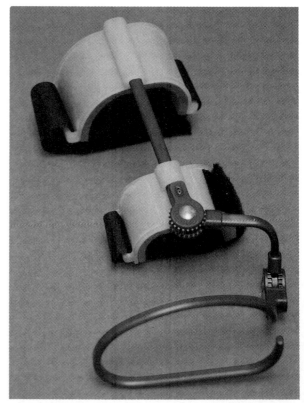

FIGURE 7–16.
A limited-motion VersaWrist splint permits functional motion without stress on articular surfaces. The range can be selected to protect selected articular surfaces. (DonJoy, Carlsbad, CA.)

control, until gentle bleeding or a strawberry surface color is observed.

The wrist is then placed in a range-limiting splint, and nonstressful motion is encouraged for 6 to 8 weeks (Fig. 7-16). Impact-loading or lifting of weights greater than 5 pounds should be avoided for 8 to 12 additional weeks.

REFERENCES

1. Poehling GG, Roth JH. Articular cartilage lesions of the wrist. In: McGinty J, ed. Operative arthroscopy. New York: Raven Press, 1991:635.
2. Watson HK, Ballet FL. The SLAC wrist: scapholunate advanced collapse pattern of degenerative arthritis. J Hand Surg [Am] 1984;9:358.
3. Salter RB, Simmonds DF, Malcolm BW, Rumble EJ, MacMichael D, Clements ND. The biological effect of continuous passive motion on the healing of full-thickness defects in articular cartilage. J Bone Joint Surg [Am] 1980;62(8):1232.
4. Ewing JW, ed. Articular cartilage and knee joint function. New York: Raven Press, 1990.

BIBLIOGRAPHY

Rogers WD, Watson HK. Radial styloid impingement after triscaphe arthrodesis. J Hand Surg [Am] 1989;14: 297.

Viegas SF. Arthroscopic treatment of osteochondritis dissecans of the scaphoid. Arthroscopy 1988;4(4):278.

Watson HK, Brenner LH. Degenerative disorders of the wrist. J Hand Surg [Am] 1985;10(6):102.

8

Triangular Fibrocartilage Complex

*T*he central disc of the triangular fibrocartilage complex (TFCC) may tear in a variety of ways, or may perforate with advancing age. Spontaneous perforation is rarely symptomatic, but any traumatic tear, regardless of age, may cause ulnar wrist pain or a clicking sensation. Palmer has developed a useful system of classifying central disc tears according to traumatic or spontaneous origin (Table 8-1).[1]

Central perforations of the disc are uncommon in people with negative ulnar variance. Chronic compression of the disc between the head of the ulna and the ulnar edge of the lunate (class IIC) is felt to be responsible for central defects (Fig 8-1). Because the ulna appears relatively longer in pronation, that is the position in which central perforations are more likely to be symptomatic.

Traumatic tears occur most commonly where the central disc is thinnest, near its attachment to the sigmoid notch of the radius (class ID; see Table 8-1). Usually linear and parallel to the sigmoid notch, these tears may curve or angulate to produce a flap of cartilage that folds with certain wrist motions (Fig. 8-2). Impingement of the flap between the ulna and the proximal carpal row may produce pain, clicking, or a sense of fullness or pressure in the wrist. Class I tears probably result from one of two mechanisms. Distal protrusion of the ulna occurs when the radius is violently loaded and is compressed in an axial direction, as in a fall on the thenar eminence. Proximal shift of the radius tears the TFCC central disc over the prominent ulnar head. Pronation increases this possibility by foreshortening the radius even further (Fig. 8-3). Fracture of the radius with shortening produces the same mechanism. In fact, class I tears of the triangular fibrocartilage (TFC) are far more commonly associated with distal radius fractures than is usually appreciated.

Tears of the central disc that parallel the ulnar or dorsal margin of the TFCC (class IB) are much less common than those previously discussed. The mechanism of injury producing these tears is unclear, although it probably involves a combination of rotation and dorsal or volar translation of the radius on the ulna. In pronation, the volar margin of the TFCC central disc and the dorsal capsule of the distal radioulnar joint (DRUJ)

Table 8—1.
CLASSIFICATION OF TRIANGULAR FIBROCARTILAGE
COMPLEX (TFCC) LESIONS

Class I: Traumatic

A. Central perforation
B. Ulnar avulsion
   with distal ulnar fracture
   without distal ulnar fracture
C. Distal avulsion
D. Radial avulsion
   with sigmoid notch fracture
   without sigmoid notch fracture

Class II: Degenerative (Ulnocarpal Abutment Syndrome)

A. TFCC wear
B. TFCC wear plus lunate and/or ulnar chondromalacia
C. TFCC perforation plus lunate and/or ulnar chondromalacia
D. TFCC perforation plus lunate and/or ulnar chondromalacia;
   plus lunotriquetral ligament perforation
E. TFCC perforation plus lunate and/or ulnar chondromalacia;
   plus lunotriquetral ligament perforation; plus ulnocarpal arthritis

Palmer AK. Triangular fibrocartilage complex lesions: a classification. J Hand Surg [Am] 1989;14(4):594.

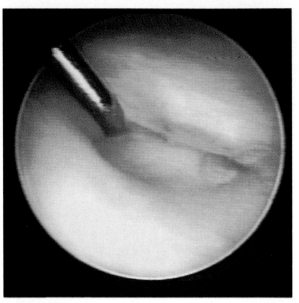

FIGURE 8—1.
A smooth, chronic, central triangular fibrocartilage complex (TFCC) perforation (right wrist) seen through the 6-U portal. Looking toward the sigmoid notch, notice the ulnar head beneath the TFCC, with apparent shortening as the wrist is held in supination. The probe is in the 4-5 portal.

are taut. The dorsal margin is lax, and the volar capsule of the DRUJ invaginates between the radius and ulna. Volar translation of the radius in this position subluxates the ulna dorsally and could be the mechanism for tearing the dorsal edge of the TFCC from the capsule or rupturing the volar radioulnar ligament (Fig. 8-4).

The opposite occurs in supination. The DRUJ capsule is lax dorsally. The dorsal margin of the TFCC is partially rolled about the ulnar styloid and is taut. Translation of the radius dorsally after supination may tear the volar triangular fibrocartilage (TFC) margin from the volar ligaments or rupture the dorsal radioulnar ligament (Fig. 8-5). Carried to an extreme, these forces could produce dorsal or volar instability of the DRUJ. Therefore, class IB and IC tears of the TFCC may be an initial stage of DRUJ instability.

CLINICAL PRESENTATION

Many tears of the TFCC central disc are well-tolerated and require no treatment. Patients with symptomatic tears of this structure complain of ill-defined, poorly localized pain on the ulnar side of

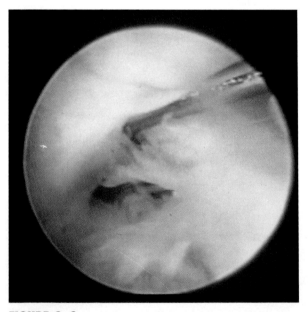

FIGURE 8—2.
Traumatic class ID tear of the triangular fibrocartilage complex viewed from the 6-R portal (right wrist). Note the avulsion from the margin of the sigmoid notch of the radius. The probe is in the 6-U portal.

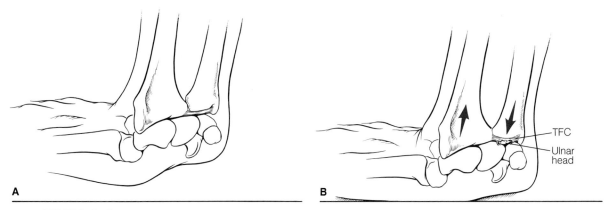

A

B

TFC

Ulnar
head

FIGURE 8–3.

Common mechanism of traumatic tears of the triangular fibrocartilage complex (TFCC). (**A**) Impact loading through the carpus displaces the radius proximally relative to the ulna. (**B**) The head of the ulna tears through the TFCC articular disc, especially in pronation, when the radius is already relatively foreshortened.

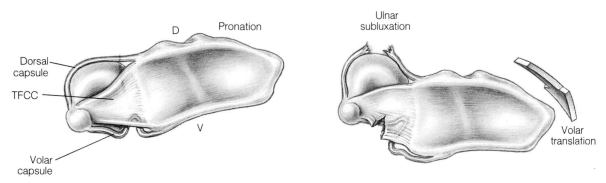

Pronation

D

Dorsal
capsule

TFCC

Volar
capsule

Ulnar
subluxation

Volar
translation

FIGURE 8–4.

The right wrist in pronation. The dorsal capsule is tight, and the volar margin of the triangular fibrocartilage complex (TFCC; the volar radioulnar ligament) is tight. Volar translation of the radius tears the volar radioulnar ligament and ruptures the dorsal distal radioulnar joint capsule, producing ulnar subluxation dorsally. D, dorsal; V, volar.

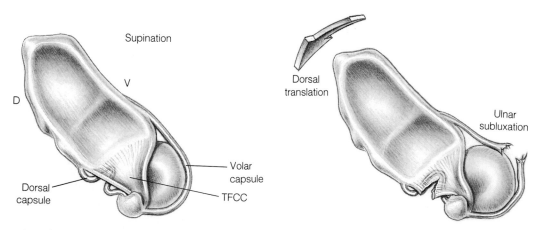

Supination

V

D

Dorsal
capsule

Volar
capsule

TFCC

Dorsal
translation

Ulnar
subluxation

FIGURE 8–5.

The right wrist in supination. The volar distal radioulnar joint (DRUJ) capsule is tight, and the dorsal margin of the triangular fibrocartilage complex (TFCC; dorsal radioulnar ligament) is tight as the dorsal margin of the radius moves farther away from the base of the ulnar styloid. Dorsal translation of the radius tears the dorsal radioulnar ligament and ruptures the volar DRUJ capsule, producing ulnar subluxation in the volar direction. D, dorsal; V, volar.

the wrist. They frequently describe the pain as deep, finding it difficult to discern between volar or dorsal location. Often they will grip the ulnar side of the wrist indicating the diffuse location of discomfort (Fig 8-6). Different positions, such as power grip, may aggravate the symptoms. Clues to the tear pattern and location can be obtained from the most provocative wrist position, but such information is not very reliable.

The presence of a clicking sensation in the wrist may be due to an unstable flap of central disc. Audible wrist clicking in pronation and supination, however, commonly comes from the extensor carpi ulnaris (ECU) tendon. The physician should be careful when interpreting clicking symptoms.

Although it is nonspecific, the most consistent and helpful physical sign of torn TFC is tenderness to palpation directly over the dorsal or volar margin of the disc. One should also evaluate the stability

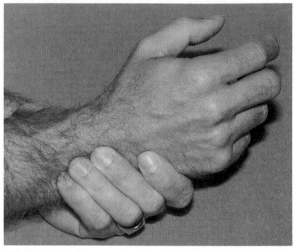

FIGURE 8–6.
Typical gesture of a patient with triangular fibrocartilage complex symptoms indicating the diffuse nature of discomfort along the ulnar side of the wrist.

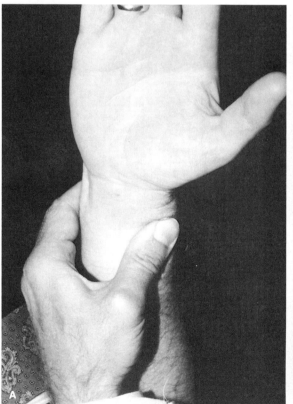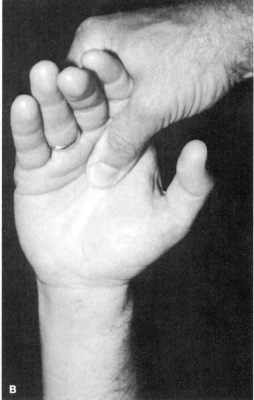

FIGURE 8–7.
(**A**) Forced passive supination applied through the forearm stresses the distal radioulnar joint and the triangular fibrocartilage complex (TFCC). (**B**) Forced passive supination or pronation applied through the hand applies more rotational stress to the carpus and may not reproduce pain associated with injury to the TFCC.

of the DRUJ by comparing passive translation between the radius and ulna in neutral rotation with that of the opposite side.

Passive pronation and supination with the examiner holding the forearm distally may cause pain if TFC is torn or if the DRUJ is unstable or arthritic. Pronation and supination force applied by gripping the hand, however, stresses the carpus more than the DRUJ or the TFCC (Fig 8-7).

Plain radiographs should be taken in neutral forearm rotation and in pronation to assess the variance in length of the radius and ulna (Figs. 8-8 and 8-9). Radial and ulnar deviation films are also helpful in evaluation of ulnocarpal abutment. None of these films are diagnostic of TFC tear; they only contribute to the examiner's clinical impression.

Arthrography is the best available imaging for

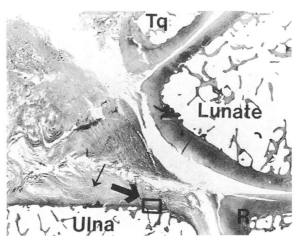

FIGURE 8—9.
A photomicroradiograph of the left wrist demonstrates ulnocarpal abutment with an attritional tear in the triangular fibrocartilage complex, as well as minimal loss of staining characteristics or thickness of the articular cartilage on the lunate. *Large arrow,* tidemark; *small arrow,* hyaline cartilage/head of ulna; R, radius; Tq, triquetrum. (Courtesy of B. Mandelbaum, M.D., Santa Monica, CA.)

confirming the diagnosis of TFC tear (Fig. 8-10). There are occasional false negative studies, as Roth has demonstrated (Fig. 8-11).[2] Tears of the TFC may be closed tightly in certain positions, preventing the flow of dye through the tear from the radiocarpal

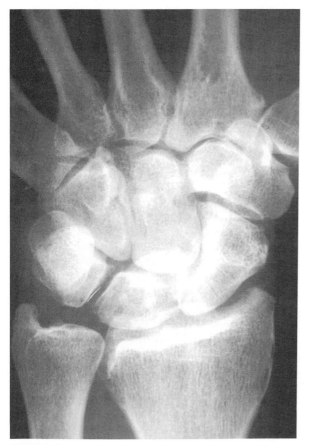

FIGURE 8—8.
Radiograph of the wrist in neutral forearm rotation showing true positive ulnar variance with ulnocarpal abutment.

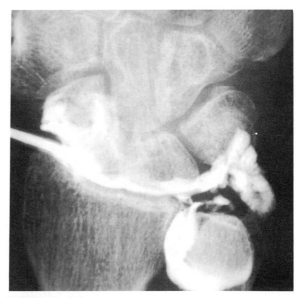

FIGURE 8—10.
This radiocarpal arthrogram of the right wrist is positive for tear of the triangular fibrocartilage complex. Note dye leaking into the distal radioulnar joint.

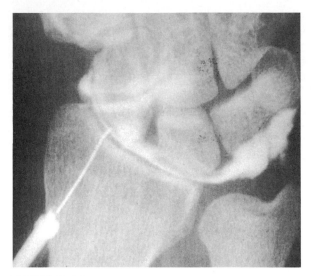

FIGURE 8–11.
This radiocarpal arthrogram is negative for tear of the triangular fibrocartilage complex. This study should be considered invalid unless confirmed by subsequent injection of the distal radioulnar joint.

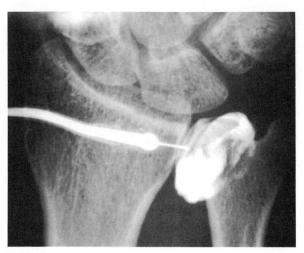

FIGURE 8–12.
This arthrogram of the distal radioulnar joint is positive for a partial thickness tear of the triangular fibrocartilage complex (proximal surface). Note the flap of cartilage indicated by a dark shadow on the inferior surface of the cartilage just above the tip of the needle.

space (see Fig. 2-30). Therefore, dye should be injected into the DRUJ if the radiocarpal injection study is negative (Fig. 8-12).

Magnetic resonance imaging is another means of imaging soft tissues but is not accurate for TFC tears because these lesions may be only a couple of millimeters in size (Fig. 8-13).

ARTHROSCOPIC APPEARANCE

The arthroscopic appearance of a torn TFCC central disc may vary depending on its thickness and the degree of degenerative changes present in the joint. Tears in thin discs have a tendency to gap open and are more easily recognized (Fig. 8-14). Thicker discs are stiffer. Even tears of significant size may lie closed and obscured unless probed and retracted (Fig. 8-15). In degenerative joints, hypertrophic synovium around the periphery can mask tears parallel to the volar or dorsal margins. Synovitis in the DRUJ may protrude through a tear, giving an appearance of ragged edges (Fig. 8-16). Degenerative discs are also slightly yellowed in comparison to adjacent articular cartilage on the lunate facet of the radius (Fig. 8-17). They also have a rougher surface texture than younger discs.

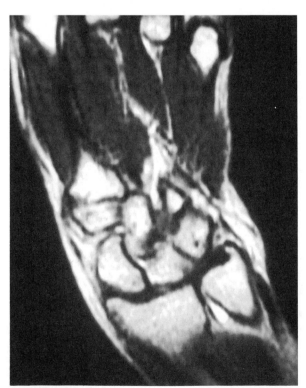

FIGURE 8–13.
This magnetic resonance imaging film of the right wrist suggests a tear of the triangular fibrocartilage complex, inferred by an altered signal from the fibrocartilage disc, and a slight change in the signal from the ulnar aspect of the lunate secondary to ulnocarpal abutment.

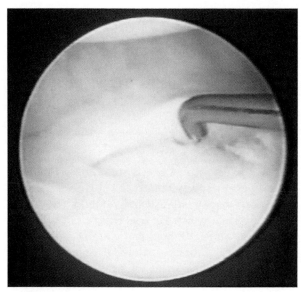

FIGURE 8–14.
A flap tear in a thin triangular fibrocartilage complex articular disc seen through the 3-4 portal (right wrist). The probe is in 4-5 portal.

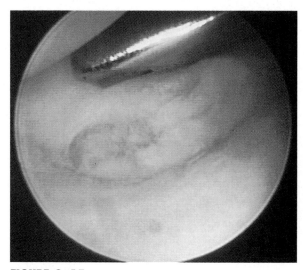

FIGURE 8–15.
A class ID tear in a thick TFCC. The tear is retracted by a shaver tip in the 6-R portal, as viewed from the 3-4 portal (right wrist).

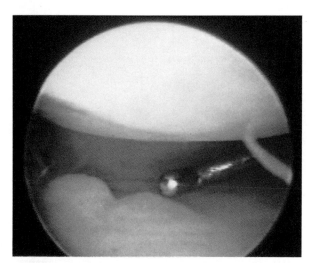

FIGURE 8–16.
An obscure triangular fibrocartilage complex tear evidenced only by synovium protruding through the tear from the distal radioulnar joint (right wrist). Viewed from the 3-4 portal; probe is in the 6-R portal.

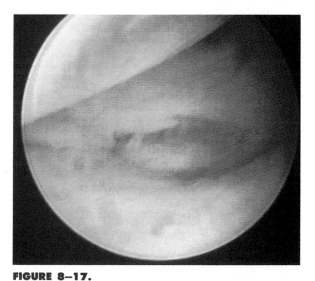

FIGURE 8–17.
A degenerative tear of the triangular fibrocartilage complex in an elderly patient. Notice the thinning and fissuring of the articular disc with yellowish discoloration on the disc (*background*) as well as on the lunate facet of the radius (*foreground*). Viewed from the 3-4 portal (right wrist).

Because some tears may not be readily visible, discs should always be probed thoroughly for defects (Fig. 8-18A). It is also helpful to briskly squeeze the dorsal and volar aspect of the DRUJ capsule, which will evert the edges of a torn TFCC as irrigating solution refluxes into the radiocarpal space (Fig 8-18B). These tears should not be confused with the prestyloid recess on the volar ulnar side of the joint, nor with the occasionally present capsular opening into the pisiform-triquetral space adjacent to the volar ulnotriquetral (UT) ligament.

Class ID TFC tears appear as linear splits ulnar to the sigmoid notch. They may vary in length from 2 to 10 mm, may be biased slightly toward the volar or dorsal side of the joint (depending on whether the injury occurred in supination or pronation), and may occasionally have an angular component at one end of the tear creating an ulnar based flap of cartilage. Probing these tears helps to define their shape and size precisely.

Class IB tears are also linear splits in the central disc, but they parallel the volar or dorsal wrist capsule. Pronation and supination can displace these tears and cause them to gap open (Fig. 8-19). On the volar side, a tear may appear as a narrow cleavage in pronation and as a spindle-shaped gap in supination. The opposite occurs on the dorsal side, with the tear narrowed in supination and opened in pronation.

TREATMENT

Not all defects in TFC require treatment. Many central perforations secondary to attrition are completely asymptomatic incidental findings and should be left alone. Small linear tears that do not gap open with wrist motion and have no unstable component are also probably best left alone. Patients should be counseled that such small tears may enlarge in the future and require treatment, but that they are just as likely not to cause further problems.

The goals of treatment of TFCC tears are to eliminate any unstable tissue by excision or repair and to minimize chances of the tear enlarging to become more severe (Fig. 8-20). Of course, remov-

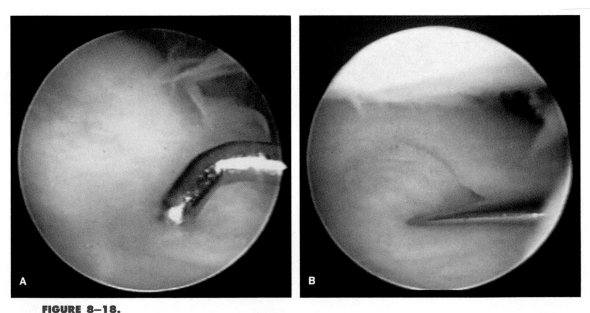

FIGURE 8—18.
(**A**) Probing examination of the triangular fibrocartilage complex (TFCC) as viewed from the 3-4 portal (right wrist). The probe is in the 6-R portal, exploring the junction of the central articular disc with the ulnotriquetral ligament in the volar direction. (**B**) Class ID tear of the TFCC. The edge of the tear is everted, and the synovium protrudes into the radiocarpal space when the distal radioulnar joint is squeezed briskly. Viewed from the 3-4 portal (right wrist).

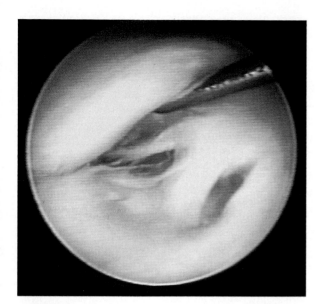

FIGURE 8—19.
A class IB tear of the triangular fibrocartilage complex (right wrist). The articular disc is avulsed from the dorsal wrist capsule. Viewed from the 3-4 portal with the needle in the 6-R portal.

fibers of the ECU tendon sheath dorsally or the volar ulnocarpal ligament volarly. The type, size, and mechanical significance of any TFCC tear can be best determined by arthroscopic examination. Excision of unstable fragments of the cartilage is also possible under arthroscopic control, and can be performed more precisely than by open techniques because of the ample light and magnification that arthroscopy provides. Arthroscopic repair of peripheral class IB tears is an experimental endeavor at this time, but may be plausible in the future. However, locating the tear exactly and preparing it arthroscopically for subsequent open repair will permit a smaller and more appropriate arthrotomy for suturing.

ing portions of the central disc raises concerns about the function of the TFCC and the deficiency that results from its injury or removal. The central cartilage disc provides a flexible articular surface to accommodate the triquetrum and a portion of the lunate. The sling must be flexible to allow rotation of the carpus about the head of the ulna. There is a debatable theory about the role of the TFCC in stabilizing the DRUJ. However, Martin and Whipple have demonstrated that excision of the entire central disc produces no instability of the joint even under rotational stress.[3] Therefore, removal of portions of the disc alters the articulation of the ulnar side of the proximal row, but seems to have no other adverse effect. If the thicker peripheral margins of the disc are intact, there will be sufficient ulnar support to cradle the convex surface of the proximal row, even in extremes of ulnar deviation, flexion, and extension. There is an apparent hoop stress support provided by the ligamentous portion of the TFCC. It is important, therefore, that these ligamentous bands remain intact. They should be inspected well before excising part of the central disc.

Access to the TFCC by way of arthrotomy is difficult. Visualization and surgical instrumentation of the cartilage is limited unless one releases the

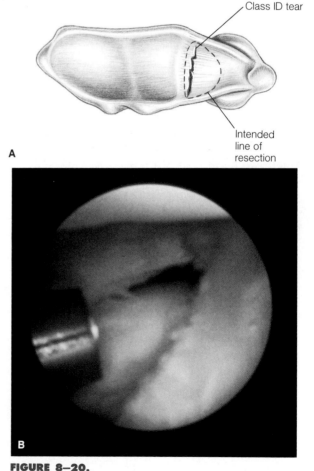

FIGURE 8—20.
(**A**) Dashed line indicates the intended contour of tissue resection for a linear class ID tear of the triangular fibrocartilage complex. (**B**) Arthroscopic photograph shows the remaining peripheral rim after resection. Note the smooth contour of the remaining fibrocartilage.

TECHNIQUE

Most TFCC tears are seen best from the 3-4 portal. Volar class IB tears are also seen best from this vantage. Dorsal class IB tears can be seen better from the 6-U portal, or, in large wrists, from the 1-2 portal. These vantage points permit visualization of dorsal tears in relation to the dorsal capsule.

For debridement of class IA or class II tears when irregular contours are present, a power shaver is the most efficient means. The shaver tip must have a relatively large opening to admit tissue from the thicker portions of the defect (Fig. 8-21). Introduced through the 6-R portal, the shaver is pressed firmly against the inner parameter of the TFC defect to excise all frayed edges. To debride the ulnar margins of the defect, it may be necessary to transfer the scope to the 6-R portal and the shaver to the 3-4 portal. Linear flap tears (class ID) should be converted to central defects (class IA). It is important to eliminate not only unstable flaps of the cartilage but also all irregular contours along the margins of the tear. Jagged margins create stress risers in the cartilage, from which new tears may progress. The finished result should leave a nearly round hole in the central disc with a diameter slightly larger than the length of the original tear.

Depending on the surgeon's preference of instruments, linear radial tears, the most common traumatic pattern, may be approached with the scope in either the 3-4 or 6-R portal. If a knife is used to excise the central portion of the disc, it should be placed through the 6-R portal with the scope in 3-4. A curved banana blade is first used to carve the volar and ulnar outline of the central excision, holding the concave surface of the blade facing proximally and radially (Fig 8-22). Then the dorsal cut is carved starting from the dorsal end of the tear facing the concave blade surface proximally. Rolling the blade to face ulnarly, the dorsal cut is advanced to meet the volar cut. Both cuts can then be deepened and completed using either the banana blade or a hooked retrograde blade. The central fragment is then removed from the joint through the 6-R portal with a grasping forceps. The inner margins should finally be trimmed with a shaver to remove any small tags of cartilage (Fig. 8-23).

Alternatively, the scope can be placed in the 6-R portal to use a suction punch or basket forceps

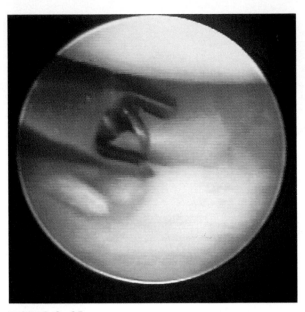

FIGURE 8—21.
A high-speed, open-end cartilage cutter (Baxter-Edwards, Santa Ana, CA) resects the central portion of the triangular fibrocartilage complex articular disc. Viewed from the 6-R portal with the cutter in the 3-4 portal.

in the 3-4 portal for piecemeal excision of the central portion of the disc (Fig. 8-24). It is usually easiest to begin this resection in the midportion of the tear where the disc is thinnest and to progress in the volar and dorsal directions. To contour the most dorsal aspect of the disc, it may be necessary to use an angulated basket forceps or to transfer the straight basket or punch to the 6-U portal. Again, the final margins should be trimmed with a shaver. These procedures can be readily performed in conjunction with reduction of fractures of the distal radius if necessary.

If the ulnar head is prominent because of positive ulnar variance or fracture shortening of the radius, and if there is significant chondromalacia on the ulnar head or any erosive change of the lunate, a leveling procedure should be considered for the ulna. Several procedures have been devised to shorten the ulna; the appropriate selection depends on the condition of the DRUJ and the amount of shortening required. In general, procedure choices include shortening the ulna shaft with plate fixation, Darrach resection of the distal ulna, Bowers' hemiresection and interposition arthroplasty, and resection

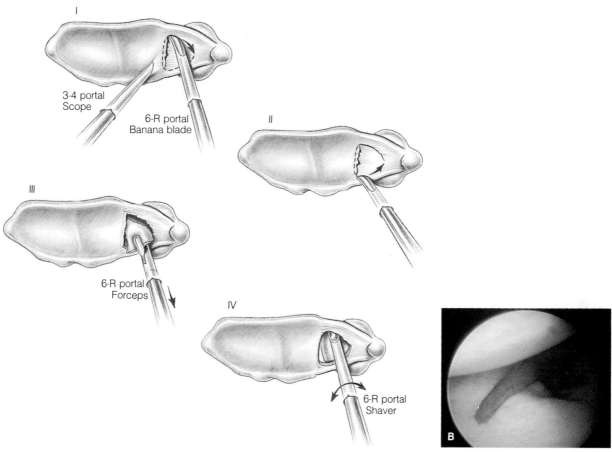

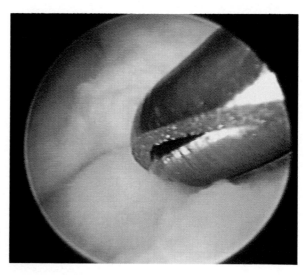

FIGURE 8–22.

(**A**) Illustration and (**B**) arthroscopic photograph of the triangular fibrocartilage complex articular disc resection using a curved banana blade (right wrist). The blade is oriented with the concave surface facing radially and proximally to begin the dorsal cut. Viewed from the 3-4 portal with the blade in the 6-R portal.

FIGURE 8–23.

A low-speed, full-radius shaver trims the remaining tags of fibrocartilage from the triangular fibrocartilage complex peripheral rim. Viewed from the 3-4 portal with the shaver in the 6-R portal (right wrist).

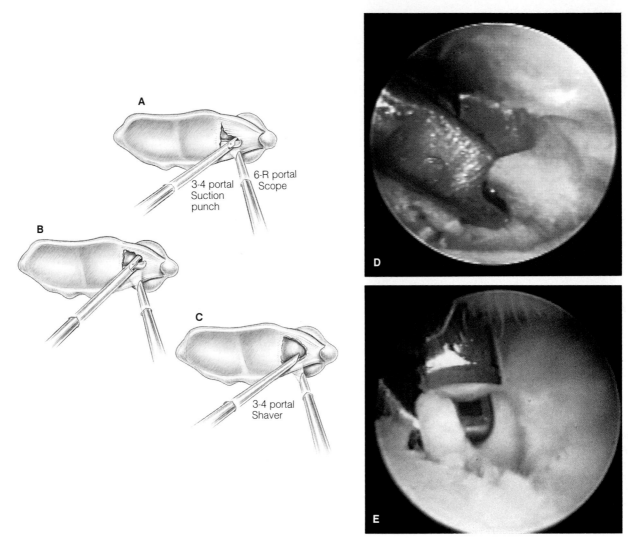

FIGURE 8—24.
Resection of the triangular fibrocartilage complex articular disc using the suction punch (Dyonics, Andover, MA) begins with the scope in the 6-R portal and a punch in the 3-4 portal. (**A**) Begin centrally, with the thinnest portion of the articular disc. (**B**) Progressively resect all unstable portions of the articular disc. (**C**) Complete the trimming process, especially the dorsal rim, with a power shaver. (**D**) Suction punch resection of the articular disc, as viewed from the 6-R portal with the punch in the 3-4 portal (right wrist). (**E**) A 45° angled basket forceps (Concept, Largo, FL) is used to complete resection of the dorsal portion of the articular disc.

of the seat of the ulna. If less than 3-mm shortening is required, and if the DRUJ function is satisfactory, resection of the ulna seat is appropriate and sufficient to decompress the ulnar side of the wrist.

This procedure can be accomplished under arthroscopic control through the defect in the TFCC. The arthroscope should be placed in the 3-4 portal. The 6-R portal is enlarged to admit a 4-mm osteo-

tome. Beginning with the wrist in supination where the ulna is relatively short, tapered slices of the ulnar head are cut to a level that is 2 to 3 mm shorter than the surface of the radius (Fig. 8-25). Each slice can be removed with a grasping forceps through the 6-R portal. Progressing around the ulnar head by gradually pronating the wrist allows resection of the entire seat of the ulna. If the TFCC defect is

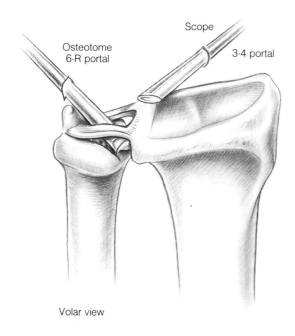

A   Volar view

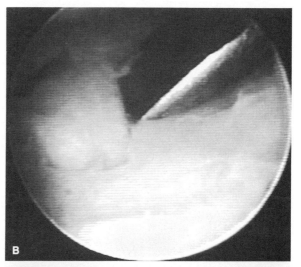

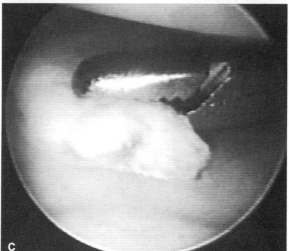

FIGURE 8–25.

(**A**) Leveling of a prominent distal ulna using an osteotome through the central defect in the triangular fibrocartilage complex (TFCC). Fragments are removed with a grasping forceps. (**B**) A ³/₁₆-inch osteotome beginning the ulna leveling procedure through the central defect in the TFCC, as viewed from the 3-4 portal (right wrist). (**C**) Removal of individual bone fragments through the 6-R portal during the ulna leveling procedure, as viewed from the 3-4 portal (right wrist).

too small to reach the most dorsal and volar portions of the ulnar seat, the scope can be moved to the 6-R portal and the osteotome to the 3-4 portal to remove the volar slice beneath the central disc in pronation. The osteotome is then placed in 6-U to remove the dorsal slice in full supination. Finally, a power burr can be used to smooth and polish the resected surface (Fig. 8-26).

It is extremely unusual for all articular cartilage to be worn off the head of the ulna from carpal abutment. In this rare circumstance, however, the entire leveling procedure can be accomplished with a power burr. An intraoperative frontal plane radiograph taken with the wrist in pronation and supi-

nation without traction is highly recommended to assess the sufficiency of the resection. The wrist should also be lavaged well with ballottement of the DRUJ to remove all loose fragments of bone. It is prudent to examine the DRUJ for loose fragments if possible.

If a class IB tear is present, an arthrotomy will be necessary to repair it. However, the arthrotomy can be minimized if the tear is freshened and trimmed smooth arthroscopically. A power shaver is ideal for this purpose. The margin of the tear should be trimmed enough to access peripheral capillaries, although active bleeding will rarely be seen.

As discussed earlier, volar tears usually close in

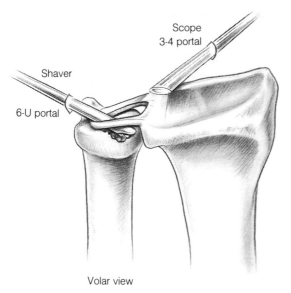

FIGURE 8–26.
Leveling of the prominent distal ulna using a burr through the 6-U portal and working through the central triangular fibrocartilage complex defect.

pronation while dorsal tears close in supination. The position in which the tear is narrowest is the best position for repair and immobilization. Once that rotational position has been determined, a 21-gauge marker needle should be placed through the ulnar capsule to enter the joint near the middle of the TFCC tear (Fig. 8-27). Then, a small arthrotomy can be made longitudinally at the needle site to access the tear for suture placement with the least possible dissection and retraction. Obviously, care must be taken to protect the ECU tendon, the flexor carpi ulnaris, and the ulnar nerve and artery.

PREFERRED METHOD

Place 8 to 10 pounds of traction on the ring and little fingers. For class IA TFCC defects requiring marginal debridement, use the technique previously described. Postoperatively, a volar plaster splint is

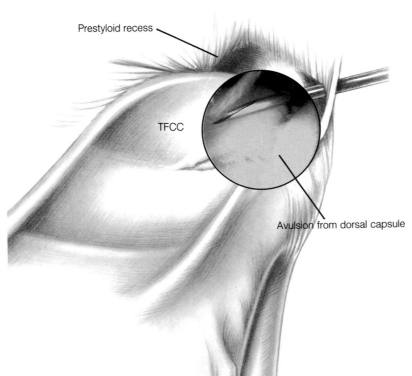

FIGURE 8–27.
A 21-gauge marker needle placed through the ulnar capsule enters the joint at the central portion of a dorsal peripheral detachment tear of the triangular fibrocartilage complex (TFCC; right wrist). Note that the tear continues as an avulsion from the dorsal aspect of the sigmoid notch.

applied for 3 days, after which time full mobilization is permitted with caution against power grip or impact loading.

For class ID tears parallel to the sigmoid notch, I prefer to resect the central portion of the disc with banana and retrograde blades. If any disc tissue remains between the tear and the radius, that tissue is resected completely to the sigmoid notch with a suction punch or with a blunt-nosed basket forceps introduced through the 6-R portal, making the defect in the central disc as round as possible. The tear is converted to a stable central defect. Postoperative care is the same as described for class IA tears.

If the ulna is prominent, the seat is resected with a 4-mm osteotome as described to level the ulna shorter than the radius in full pronation. With ulnar prominence, a generous resection of the central disc is performed to provide maximum decompression of the ulnar side without compromising peripheral support for the proximal row. The same postoperative splinting is used for 7 days because of additional surgical trauma and the enlarged portals. Pronation and supination are permitted immediately, however.

For peripheral detachment tears, the procedure previously described is preferred. The arthrotomy rarely requires more than a 15-mm skin incision. The defect in the TFC is sutured with 4–0 braided nonabsorbable suture, using a small, sturdy cleft palate needle. Subcuticular skin closure is reinforced with sterile tapes, and a sugar-tong splint is applied in the position determined to best narrow the tear edges. Motion is allowed after 4 weeks but without stress or grip strengthening for 3 months following the procedure.

CLINICAL RESULTS

Patients treated in this manner for TFCC tears have fared exceptionally well. Pain relief has been predictably good, although not always complete. There have been no adverse sequelae resulting from trimming central tears or resecting the central portion of the disc for linear radial tears, nor has there been any noticeable loss of motion. Discomfort may persist following the leveling procedure for as long as 6 months, although it gradually subsides. Slight loss of supination has been observed, although the reason for this loss is unknown.

Experience with repair of peripheral class 1B tears is limited. These tears are not common. Results have ranged from pain-free resumption of throwing sports to persistent slight pain. We have observed up to a 20° loss of supination. Care should always be taken to protect the cutaneous branches of the ulnar nerve when an arthrotomy is made, and to securely close the floor of the ECU tendon sheath when it is incised to repair dorsal tears.

REFERENCES

1. Palmer AK. Triangular fibrocartilage complex lesions: a classification. J Hand Surg [Am] 1989;14(4):594.
2. Roth JH, Haddad RG. Radiocarpal arthroscopy and arthrography in the diagnosis of ulnar wrist pain. Arthroscopy 1986;2(4):234.
3. Martin DR, Whipple TL, Yates CK. The role of the triangular fibrocartilage complex in distal radioulnar joint stability: a cadaver study. J Hand Surg [Am] (in press).

BIBLIOGRAPHY

Boulas HJ, Milek MA. Ulnar shortening for tears of the triangular fibrocartilaginous complex. J Hand Surg [Am] 1990;15(3):415.

Brown DE, Lichtman DM. The evalutation of chronic wrist pain. Orthop Clin North Am 1984;15(2):183.

Green DP. The sore wrist without a fracture. Inst Course Lect 1985;34:300.

King GJ, McMurtry RY, Rubenstein JD, Gertzbein SB. Kinematics of the distal radioulnar joint. J Hand Surg [Am] 1986;11(6):798.

Menon J, Wood VE, Schoene HR, Frykman GK, Hohl JC, Bestard EA. Isolated tears of the triangular fibrocartilage of the wrist: results of partial excision. J Hand Surg [Am] 1984;9(4):527.

Mizuseki T, Watari S, Ishida O, Ikuta Y. A case report of isolated traumatic tear of the triangular fibrocartilage. Hiroshima J Med Sci 1986;35(1):63.

Nevaiser RJ, Palmer AK. Traumatic perforation of the articular disc of the triangular fibrocartilage complex of the wrist. Bull Hosp J Dis Orthop Inst 1984;44(2):376.

Palmer AK. The distal radioulnar joint. Anatomy, biomechanics, and triangular fibrocartilage complex abnormalities. Hand Clin 1987;3(1):31.

Palmer AK. Triangular fibrocartilage complex lesions: a classification. J Hand Surg [Am] 1989;14(4):594.

Palmer AK, Werner FW, Glisson RR, Murphy DJ. Partial

excision of the triangular fibrocartilage complex. J Hand Surg [Am] 1988;13(3):391.

Palmer AK, Werner FW. The triangular fibrocartilage complex of the wrist—anatomy and function. J Hand Surg [Am] 1981;6(2):153.

Quinn SF, Belsole RS, Greene TL, Rayhack JM. Work in progress: postarthrography computed tomography of the wrist: evaluation of the traingular fibrocartilage complex. Skeletal Radiol 1989:17(8):565.

Roth JH, Haddad RG. Radiocarpal arthroscopy and arthrography in the diagnosis of ulnar wrist pain. Arthroscopy 1986;2(4):234.

Trumble T, Glisson RR, Seaber AV, Urbaniak JR. Forearm force transmission after surgical treatment of distal radioulnar joint disorders. J Hand Surg [Am] 1987; 12(2):196.

van der Linden AJ. Disk lesion of the wrist joint. J Hand Surg [Am] 1986;11(4):490.

Weigl K, Spira E. The traingular fibrocartilage of the wrist joint. Reconstr Surg Traumatol 1969;11:139.

Werner FW, Glisson RR, Murphy DJ, Palmer AK. Force transmission through the distal radioulnar carpal joint: effect of ulnar lengthening and shortening. Handchir Mikrochir Plast Chir 1986;18(5):304.

9

Intrinsic Ligaments
and Carpal Instability

*T*he intrinsic ligaments of the wrist connect the bones within the proximal and distal carpal rows. While they work in concert with the extrinsic capsular ligaments, their primary functions are to prevent separation of the carpals during axial loading and to limit translational movements between these bones in the sagittal plane. The intrinsic ligaments of the proximal carpal row separate the midcarpal space from the radiocarpal space (Fig. 9-1). The fibers of these ligaments attach to the edges of the proximal articular surfaces of the proximal row. Their fibers blend with the hyaline cartilage of the proximal row and merge into the dorsal and volar capsules distally (Fig. 9-2).

The scapholunate ligament is slightly longer than the lunotriquetral ligament to accommodate the greater degree of flexion and extension between the scaphoid and lunate. Dissections by the author indicate that the volar portions of both ligaments are thicker than the dorsal aspect. The scapholunate ligament is thicker at its scaphoid attachment and the lunotriquetral ligament is thicker at the lunate attachment. Therefore, when these ligaments tear, it is usually through the thinner ulnar aspect.

During axial loading of the wrist, the capitate and hamate wedge into the concave acetabular surface of the proximal row. As loading forces are distributed radially on the surface of the capitate, the intrinsic ligaments tighten. The proximal aspect of the intercarpal spaces between scaphoid and lunate and between lunate and triquetrum open slightly, but the distal surfaces of these articulations are compressed, effectively tightening the proximal row around the convex surface of the capitate and hamate (Fig. 9-3). Without intact intrinsic ligaments, the integrity of the acetabulum of the proximal row would be lost, and the ability of the wrist to accommodate axial load would be reduced, especially in eccentric positions.

SCAPHOLUNATE DISSOCIATION

Injuries to the scapholunate ligament can result from extreme flexion, hyperextension, or violent axial loading. As the wrist flexes, the scaphoid

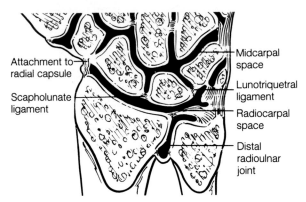

FIGURE 9–1.

Intrinsic intercarpal ligaments define the midcarpal space. Note that none of these ligaments would be visible arthroscopically between the proximal and distal rows.

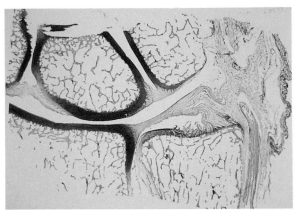

FIGURE 9–2.

Photomicrograph (whole mount, right wrist) showing the scapholunate and lunotriquetral ligament fibers merging with hyaline cartilage of the respective carpal bones. (Safranin-O stain; courtesy of S.P. Arnoczky, D.V.M., Dipl. A.C.V.S., New York, NY.)

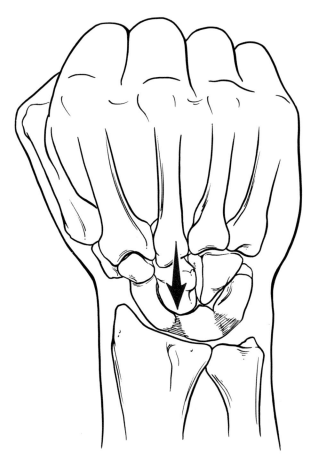

FIGURE 9–3.

Axial load on the carpus of a clenched fist causes the capitate and hamate to wedge into the proximal row. This produces compression of the intercarpal spaces of the proximal row distally, and distraction with tension on the intrinsic ligaments proximally.

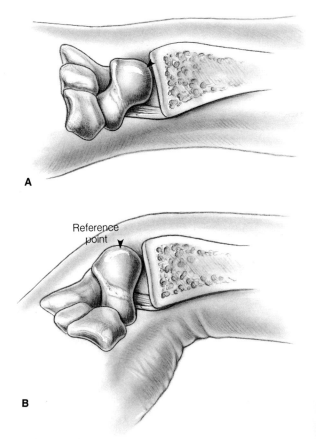

FIGURE 9–4.

(**A**) Lateral projection of the right wrist in neutral position. (**B**) In wrist flexion, the trapezium and trapezoid shift dorsally on the scaphoid as it flexes over the volar radioscaphocapitate ligament. This creates a mechanical lever that displaces the proximal pole of the scaphoid dorsally relative to the radius.

rotates in a volar direction and its articulation with the trapezium and trapezoid shifts dorsally (Fig. 9-4). Axial loading on the radial side of the wrist applies an additional flexion force to the scaphoid. Pivoting about the volar radioscaphocapitate (RSC) ligament, the long scaphoid becomes a mechanical lever, and its proximal pole is displaced dorsally. Here the thinner portion of the scapholunate ligament may tear.

A similar effect may occur when the wrist is loaded axially in radial deviation. Here again the scaphoid is flexed, and the wedge effect of the capitate and hamate forces the scaphoid and lunate apart, tearing the intrinsic ligament. Hyperextension of the wrist can rupture the volar RSC ligament (Fig. 9-5). The scaphoid moves with the distal carpal row, tearing away from the lunate. Losing its volar ligamentous support, the scaphoid then collapses into flexion when the wrist returns to neutral (Fig. 9-6).

Lesser injuries to the scapholunate ligament may

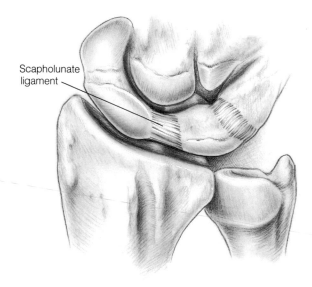

FIGURE 9–5.
An anteroposterior projection of the right wrist in extension shows the scaphoid oriented longitudinally and separating from the lunate, putting strain on the scapholunate ligament.

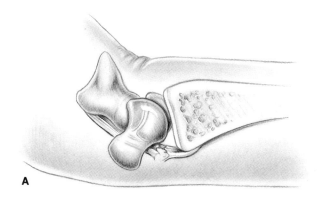

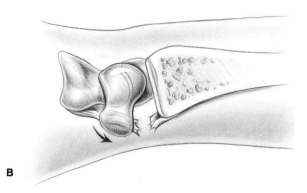

FIGURE 9–6.
Rupture of the volar radioscaphocapitate (RSC) ligament. (**A**) Hyperextension of the wrist ruptures the RSC ligament between the radius and capitate, disabling the volar support of the scaphoid. (**B**) As the wrist returns to neutral position, the scaphoid is allowed to collapse passively into flexion.

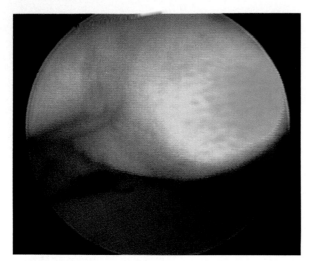

FIGURE 9–7.
Stretch injury to the scapholunate ligament as viewed from the 3-4 portal (right wrist). The prominent contour of the lunate is caused by dorsal intercalated segmental instability posturing while the lunate rotates into flexion.

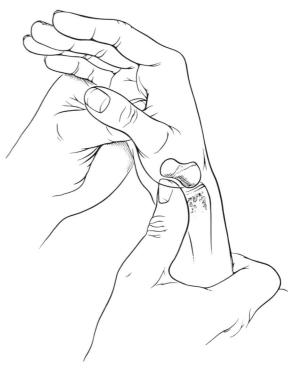

FIGURE 9–8.
Watson's test for scapholunate dissociation. The examiners's thumb prevents the scaphoid from flexing while the wrist is passively flexed or deviated radially.

only stretch the fibers, elongating the ligament enough to increase motion between the scaphoid and lunate (Fig. 9-7). Increased motion can produce pain and subluxation of the proximal poles of the scaphoid. Ultimately, it may cause degenerative change on the articular surfaces of the scaphoid and radius. There will be no discernible increase in the space between scaphoid and lunate on plain radiographs, and the arthrogram will be essentially normal. The Watson test may be positive, however. In this test, the examiner blocks scaphoid flexion by applying pressure to the distal volar scaphoid tubercle, and then passively flexes or radially deviates the wrist (Fig. 9-8). This maneuver will cause pain or a palpable shift of the scaphoid as the proximal pole subluxates dorsally.

In more severe injuries to the scapholunate ligament, the fibers are actually ruptured or avulsed from their insertion on the lunate. Symptoms may be no more severe than in cases of stretch injury, depending on the stressful activities to which the wrist is subjected.

Plain radiographs may show an increase in the space between the scaphoid and lunate. At greater extremes this finding is known as the Terry Thomas sign (Fig. 9-9). An arthrogram will usually demonstrate communication between the radiocarpal

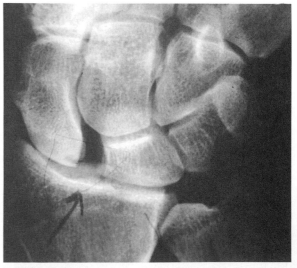

FIGURE 9–9.
The Terry Thomas sign. This right wrist with scapholunate dissociation manifests a large gap in the proximal carpal row (*arrow*).

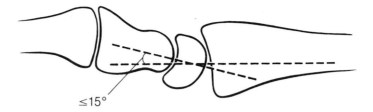

FIGURE 9—10.

A method of measuring the radiolunate angle. The lunate axis is represented by a line bisecting its distal concave surface in the lateral projection.

and midcarpal spaces. False-negative studies may occur, however, if the defect is small and the pressure of injecting the radiocarpal space closes a flap of the torn ligament and seals the communication. When there is high clinical suspicion that the scaphoid and lunate may be dissociated, but the radiocarpal injection initially reveals no communication between the radiocarpal and midcarpal spaces, the wrist should be exercised under fluoroscopic control in an attempt to open the tear briefly and allow dye to flow across the defect. If this fails, a second injection into the midcarpal space (once the original contrast medium has been absorbed) will more likely open the scapholunate ligament defect and reveal communication between the two spaces.

Besides widening of the scapholunate interval, other signs of scapholunate dissociation may be found on plain radiographs. On the lateral projection, the orientation of the lunate normally is governed by its attachment to the scaphoid and to the triquetrum. The scaphoid exerts a flexion influence on the lunate while the triquetrum exerts an extension influence. Disruption of the scapholunate ligament leaves the extension influence of the triquetrum unbalanced and causes the lunate to tilt into extension (dorsal intercalated segmental instability; DISI). On the lateral radiograph, this dorsal tilt may be appreciated. It can be accentuated by obtaining a clenched-fist view to compress the scaphoid and lunate. More than a 15° dorsal angulation of the lunate with respect to the shaft of the radius is considered abnormal (Fig. 9-10).

Similarly, the scapholunate angle can be measured on the lateral projection as the angle between the axis of the scaphoid and the orientation of the lunate (Fig. 9-11). Scapholunate angles greater than 70° are considered abnormal, reflecting excessive passive flexion of the scaphoid. This finding is more likely to occur when the volar RSC ligament has also been stretched or torn so that there is little volar support.

Still another suggestive radiographic sign of scapholunate dissociation is the "ring sign." The ring sign is formed by the cortical rim of the distal pole of the scaphoid seen on the posteroanterior projection when the scaphoid is excessively flexed. The ring sign cannot be measured or otherwise quantified, and can occur as a false positive if the wrist is slightly pronated relative to the x-ray beam.

Arthroscopic Appearance

Disruption of the scapholunate interval is best seen arthroscopically by examining the ligament from the 3-4 portal of the radiocarpal space. The ligament can be palpated with a probe in the 4-5 portal. Normally it has a glistening appearance that blends imperceptibly with the articular cartilage of the scaphoid and lunate to either side. The only visual clue to its presence in young healthy individuals is a reversal of the convex contour of the proximal row between the scaphoid and lunate. When palpating the ligament, the wrist can be flexed and extended to see the more dorsal and volar aspects. Look for fibrillation of the fibers on the ligament surface and for redundancy or folding of the ligament, especially with extension and ulnar deviation.

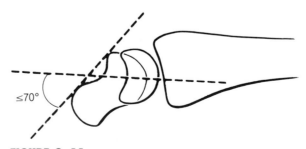

FIGURE 9—11.

A method of measuring the scapholunate angle in the lateral projection.

If the ligament is disrupted, see if the scapholunate interval can be reduced normally. Also look for signs of articular degeneration on the proximal pole of the scaphoid and the scaphoid facet of the radius.

In the midcarpal space, abnormal diastasis between the scaphoid and lunate will be more apparent. There are no intrinsic ligaments present in the midcarpal space. The edges of the articulation between scaphoid and lunate are clearly visible. The intercarpal gap between scaphoid and lunate can be compared with that between the lunate and triquetrum and should appear similar. Flexion or radial deviation of the wrist may accentuate an abnormally wide scapholunate interval. Chronic cases of scapholunate dissociation, even if mild, will cause fibrillated cartilage changes along the articular margins of the scaphoid and lunate adjacent to the scapholunate interval. This probably reflects shearing forces when these edges are compressed during axial load. These changes reflect abnormal wear patterns in an area of incongruent articulation.

On the volar aspect of the midcarpal space, the articular margins of the scaphoid and lunate should align perfectly in neutral wrist position (Fig. 9-12). Dorsal pressure on the lunate or scaphoid normally does not produce translational motion between these carpals. Radial deviation should cause no more than a millimeter dip in the volar scaphoid margin relative to the lunate. A small diameter C-wire or K-wire can be drilled into the lunate dorsally to be used as a joystick for manipulation of this carpal. With experience, one will soon appreciate normal ranges of scapholunate motion viewed in the midcarpal space.

Treatment Options

No treatment approach has been proved the best for either acute or chronic scapholunate dissociation. This condition may progress with time to a well-recognized degenerative pattern commonly referred to as the scapholunate advanced collapse (SLAC) wrist.[1,2] The SLAC wrist consists of degenerative arthritis between the radial styloid and the proximal pole of the scaphoid, disintegrated motion between the scaphoid and lunate, and degenerative changes in the midcarpal space between the lunate and capitate. The lunate may shift in a volar ulnar direction allowing the capitate to migrate proximally and dorsally. This condition can be extremely debilitating, but the instances in which it will develop are not predictable. If SLAC wrist patterns can be averted by reasonable means through timely treatment of scapholunate dissociation, it would be highly beneficial.

Treatment options for scapholunate instability include functional bracing, ligament repair, ligament reconstruction with tendon grafts, scapholunate fusion, scaphotrapeziotrapezoid (STT; triscaphe) fusion and scaphocapitate fusion. Either of the intercarpal fusions that link the proximal and distal rows will limit wrist motion significantly. In addition, they concentrate load-bearing forces on the radioscaphoid articulation where arthrosis is likely to develop as a result of chronic scapholunate instability. Fusion of the scapholunate joint is difficult to achieve. The articular surface is small, loading forces distract the surfaces, and resection of the articular cartilage and subcondylar bone widens the scapholunate gap even further.

Neither ligament reconstruction nor repair have proven to be durable solutions, and the surgical approach necessary for these procedures is rather extensive. Long-term functional bracing requires an extremely cooperative and tolerant patient. The

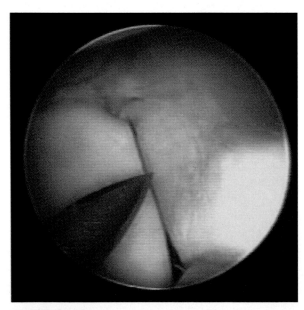

FIGURE 9–12.
Midcarpal space (right wrist) showing perfectly aligned articulation between scaphoid (*left*) and lunate (*right*).

limitations imposed by an external appliance on the hand is considerable. Attempts have been made in the past to reduce the scaphoid under fluoroscopy and pin it in place in hopes of restoring stability to the scapholunate interval. However, the chances of the thin intrinsic scapholunate healing in midsubstance or reattaching to the lunate spontaneously are small. This approach has generally been unsuccessful.

Preferred Method

Because each treatment option discussed above for scapholunate instability has produced suboptimal results, I have attempted to treat this disorder in a relatively conservative manner. A fibrous ankylosis can be induced between the scaphoid and lunate by placing multiple K-wires across this interval after achieving anatomic reduction under arthroscopic control (Fig. 9-13).

Technique

Using regional or general anesthesia, traction is applied to the wrist through the index and long

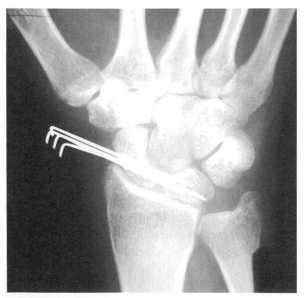

FIGURE 9–13.
The right wrist after arthroscopic reduction and multiple pin fixation of the scapholunate joint. Note that the pins do not violate any other articular surface.

fingers. The radiocarpal space is inspected arthroscopically through the 3-4 portal. K-wires are inserted through the radial joint capsule using a small-diameter skin cannula or a 16-gauge hypodermic needle just radial to the extensor carpi radialis longus (ECRL) tendon. Under direct vision, two K-wires are drilled into the proximal pole of the scaphoid aimed toward the lunate. The arthroscope is then transferred to the RMC portal to inspect the midcarpal space. The scaphoid is reduced to the lunate by placing the wrist in slight extension and ulnar deviation, by manipulating the two pins placed in the scaphoid, or by manipulating an additional pin that may be placed in the lunate dorsally. When reduced, the carpals are transfixed by advancing the pins through the scaphoid into the lunate. A total of 4 to 5 pins are placed across this interval using arthroscopy and intraoperative radiographs to assure that the articular surfaces of the radiocarpal and midcarpal spaces are not violated. The pins are bent, cut short, and left protruding through the skin.

A thumb spica cast is applied, and the pin tracks are inspected and cleaned through a cast window at 2-week intervals. Depending on the status of the pin tracks, the chronicity of the instability, and the width of diastasis between the scaphoid and lunate, the pins are left in place 6 to 8 weeks. They can be removed without anesthesia. The wrist is splinted with a cock-up wrist splint or limited-range brace for an additional 4 weeks.

This technique has proven effective in restoring scapholunate stability in over 80% of cases with up to 4 years follow-up.[3] Success is more predictable if the instability is less than 3 months old and if there is minimal or no diastasis between the scaphoid and lunate. Larger degrees of diastasis reflect an associated injury to the volar RSC ligament, depriving the scaphoid of crucial volar support. Such cases cannot be well-managed by ankylosis of the scapholunate interval alone.

LUNOTRIQUETRAL LIGAMENT INSTABILITY

As in the case of the scapholunate ligament, the lunotriquetral ligament is short, spanning the interval between the lunate and triquetrum from dorsal to volar. The ligament becomes confluent with the hyaline cartilage of the proximal articular surface of the lunate and triquetrum and merges with the fibers of the dorsal and volar capsules. It controls spread of the interval between these two carpal bones as well as translational movement anterior and posterior.

The lunotriquetral ligament is thicker volar than dorsal, and is thicker at its lunate attachment than it is at the attachment to the triquetrum.

Injuries to the lunotriquetral ligament may occur with extremes of forceful pronation or with extreme dorsally directed forces on the pisiform, such as a fall on the palmar ulnar aspect of the outstretched hand. In this latter mechanism, the pisiform articulation with the triquetrum forces the triquetrum dorsally, tearing it away from the lunate.

The lunotriquetral ligament may be irreversibly stretched, or can rupture completely. Frequently it is avulsed from its weaker attachment to triquetrum. Injury to the lunotriquetral ligament may represent a continuum of injury to the volar ulnocarpal ligaments. Specifically, as the volar ulnotriquetral (UT) ligament supporting the ulnar side of the wrist is torn with hyperpronation or extension, the triquetrum gains additional anterior and posterior mobility with respect to the lunate. The lunotriquetral ligament then will tear as the pronation or extension force continues (Fig. 9-14).

Midcarpal instability (MCI) is partially the result of injury to the volar triquetro-hamate-capitate (THC) ligament. This ligament is an extension of the volar UT ligament and can be injured by a similar loading pattern (Fig. 9-15). This helps to explain the common association of MCI with lunotriquetral instability and tears of the lunotriquetral ligament.

Patients presenting with symptomatic tears of the lunotriquetral ligament usually localize their discomfort in the dorsal ulnar aspect of the wrist. It may be exacerbated by passive pronation of the hand on the fixed forearm or by loading the palmar ulnar side of the wrist in extension (as in performing a push-up). If MCI is also present, there may be a palpable or visible shift of the proximal carpal row if the patient is asked to clench the fist in pronation and then deviate the hand to the ulnar side (Fig. 9-16).

Localized tenderness over the lunotriquetral interval is common, but significant lunotriquetral instability is marked by the presence of pain when the ulnar side of the triquetrum is compressed just distal

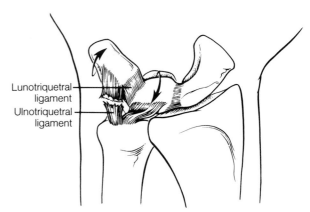

Lunotriquetral ligament
Ulnotriquetral ligament

FIGURE 9–14.

Hyperextension or hyperpronation forces can tear the volar ulnotriquetral ligament. Continuation of these forces may tear the intrinsic lunotriquetral ligament. Lunotriquetral instability is manifest by dorsal intercalary segment instability posturing of the lunate and by malalignment of the distal articular surface of the proximal carpal row.

to the ulnar styloid (see Fig. 2-15). The examiner may also reproduce pain or appreciate excessive motion with the Shuck test (see Fig. 2-14). In this maneuver, the examiner holds the triquetrum and pisiform with one hand, the lunate with the other, and attempts to translate the lunate and triquetrum in alternating volar and dorsal directions.

Radiographs may show an unusually wide gap between the lunate and triquetrum, or a step-off in the convex contour of the proximal carpal row. Comparison films of the opposite wrist should be obtained if there is any doubt about the integrity of the lunotriquetral joint. An arthrogram performed under fluoroscopic control will show contrast medium passing through the lunotriquetral interval. The contrast medium may be injected into the radiocarpal space or the midcarpal space, but a midcarpal injection is more reliable because of the possible valve effect with certain ligament tears as discussed above. Plain films in a lateral projection will often demonstrate volar angulation of the lunate caused by the flexion influence of the scaphoid with loss of the extension counterbalance of the triquetrum. This volar tilt posture of the lunate is commonly referred to as volar intercalated segmental instability (VISI) pattern.

Treatment of complex instability patterns on the ulnar side of the wrist usually entails tightening or reconstruction of the volar carpal ligaments, possibly combined with dorsal capsulorrhaphy to reduce the volar tilt of the lunate. If arthrosis is present in the

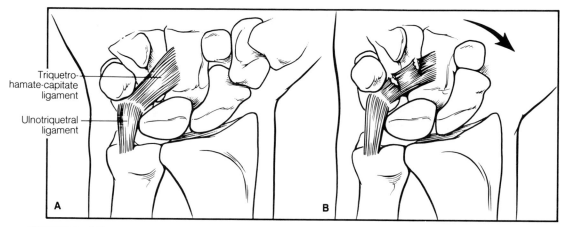

FIGURE 9–15.

Hyperextension or combined excessive radial deviation and extension can tear the volar triquetro-hamate-capitate ligament, producing midcarpal instability. (**A**) Neutral anatomic position. (**B**) Extension with radial deviation.

midcarpal space, a four-corner arthrodesis between capitate, hamate, triquetrum, and lunate may be preferable. For simpler forms of ulnar carpal instability involving only the lunate and triquetrum, it may be possible to preserve more motion by fusing only the lunotriquetral interval. Even so, solid lunotriquetral arthrodesis may be difficult to achieve, and it inevitably sacrifices some degree of motion.

Preferred Treatment

Again, in an effort to restore the integrity of the proximal carpal row with the least possible surgical insult, and to maintain as much wrist motion as possible, I prefer to treat isolated lunotriquetral instability with arthroscopic reduction and multiple pin fixation. In all acute lesions of the lunotriquetral

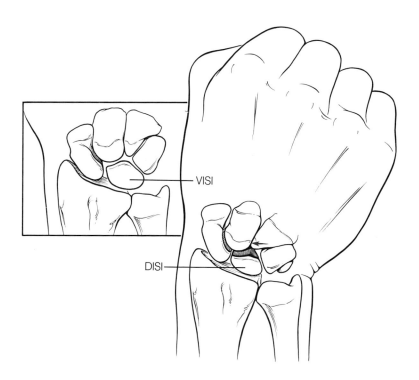

FIGURE 9–16.

The midcarpal shift (''catch-up clunk'') in midcarpal instability. With a closed fist in pronation, the hand is deviated ulnarward. The lunate is pinned in a volar intercalary segment instability (VISI) position by the proximal pole of the hamate, then it shifts suddenly to a dorsal intercalary segment instability (DISI) posture as the proximal pole of hamate crosses the lunotriquetral interval.

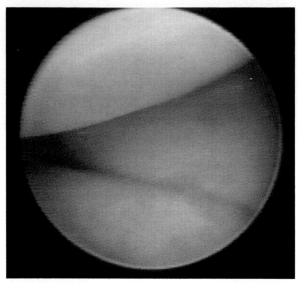

FIGURE 9–17.
Precisely reduced lunotriquetral interval seen through the midcarpal space from the radial midcarpal portal (right wrist). Note that the volar articular corners of the lunate and triquetrum are aligned evenly, and the lunotriquetral margins are parallel.

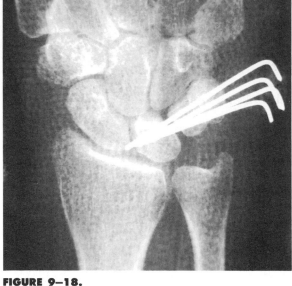

FIGURE 9–18.
Radiograph of right wrist after arthroscopic reduction and internal fixation of lunotriquetral instability.

ligament or chronic tears with little or no diastasis between the lunate and triquetrum, a controlled fibrous ankylosis can be induced that will usually restore and maintain the integrity of the proximal carpal row.

Fingertrap traction is applied to the little and ring fingers, with the wrist positioned in slight flexion and radial deviation to help reduce the triquetrum to the lunate. With the arthroscope in the 4-5 or 6-R portal, the remains of the lunotriquetral ligament can be trimmed and freshened with a suction punch, basket forceps, or shaver through the 6-U portal. Using small skin cannulae or 16-gauge hypodermic needles to protect the cutaneous branches of the ulnar nerve, small K-wires are introduced into the triquetrum adjacent to the extensor carpi ulnaris (ECU) tendon, aiming toward the lunate. The arthroscope is then transferred to the RMC portal. The lunotriquetral interval is reduced anatomically, paying particular attention to the distal volar margins of these carpals (Fig. 9-17). The wires are then advanced across the lunotriquetral interval into the lunate. A total of 4 or 5 wires are introduced with their position confirmed by intraoperative radiographs (Fig. 9-18).

The pins are bent and cut short. A short arm cast is applied for 6 to 8 weeks, with pin tracks tended every 10 to 14 days through a cast window. When the pins are removed after 6 to 8 weeks, a protective wrist splint is worn for an additional month. Patients are cautioned against impact loading or forceful rotational movements of the wrist for 3 additional months.

Experience with this technique is limited to 4 years follow-up at the time of this writing. Close review of our patient series, however, reveals better than 80% good results with arthroscopic reduction and internal fixation (ARIF) of the lunotriquetral interval based on pain relief, grip strength, maintenance of a closed lunotriquetral interval by radiography and subjective wrist stability.

REFERENCES

1. Watson HK, Black DM. Instabilities of the wrist. Hand Clin 1987;3(1):103.
2. Watson HK, Brenner LH. Degenerative disorders of the wrist. J Hand Surg [Am] 1985;10(6):1002.
3. Whipple TL, Schengel D, Caffrey D, Ellis F. Treat-

ment of scapholunate dissociation by arthroscopic reduction and internal fixation. Presented at the International Wrist Investigators' Workshop, Long Beach, California, May 1990.

BIBLIOGRAPHY

Belsole RJ, Hilbelink D, Llewellyn JA, Dale M, Stenzler S, Rayhack JM. Scaphoid orientation and location from computed three dimensional carpal models. Orthop Clin North Am 1986;17(3):510.

Frykman E. Dislocation of the triquetrum: case report. Scand J Plast Reconstr Surg 1980;14(2):205.

Garcia-Elias M, Dobyns JH, Cooney WP III, Linscheid RL. Traumatic axial dislocations of the carpus. J Hand Surg (Am) 1989;14(3):446.

Griffiths H, Jacobs J, Torre B. Wrist injuries and instability. Orthopedics 1986;9(1):94.

Hastings DE, Silver RL. Intercarpal arthrodesis in the management of chronic carpal instability after trauma. J Hand Surg [Am] 1984;9(6):834.

Jackson WT, Protas JM. Snapping scapholunate subluxation. J Hand Surg [Am] 1981;6(6):590.

Jasmine MS, Packer JW, Edwards GS Jr. Irreducible transcaphoid perilunate dislocation. J Hand Surg [Am] 1988;13(2):212.

Kleimman WB. Management of chronic rotary subluxation of the scaphoid by scaphotrapeziotrapezoid arthrodesis: rationale for the technique, post-operative changes in biomechanics and results. Hand Clin 1987;3(1):113.

Lichtman DM. Management of chronic rotary subluxation of the scaphoid by scaphotrapeziotrapezoid arthrodesis (letter). J Hand Surg [Am] 1983;8(2):223.

Linscheid RL, Dobyns JH. The unified concept of carpal injuries. Ann Chir Main 1984;3(1):35.

Logan SE, Nowak MD, Gould PL, Weeks PM. Biomechanical behavior of the scapholunate ligaments. Biomed Sci Instrum 1986:81.

Logan SE, Nowak MD. Intrinsic and extrinsic wrist ligaments: biomechanical and functional differences. Biomed Sci Instrum 1987;23:9.

Mayfield JK. Patterns of injury to carpal ligaments: a spectrum. Clin Orthop 1984;187:36.

Panting AL, Lamb DW, Noble J, Haw CS. Dislocations of the lunate with and without fracture of the scaphoid. J Bone Joint Surg [Br] 1984;66(3):391.

Penny WH III, Green TL. Volar radiocarpal dislocation with ulnar translocation. J Orthop Trauma 1988;2(4):322.

Pin PG, Nowak M, Logan SE, Young VL, Gilula LA, Weeks PM. Coincident rupture of the scapholunate and lunotriquetral ligaments without perilunate dislocation: pathomechanics and management. J Hand Surg [Am] 1990;15(1):110.

Pin PG, Young VL, Gilula LA, Weeks PM. Management of chronic lunotriquetral ligament tears. J Hand Surg [Am] 1989;14(1):77.

Siegert JJ, Frassica FJ, Amadio PC. Treatment of chronic perilunate dislocations. J Hand Surg [Am] 1988;13(2):206.

Taleisnik J. Classification of carpal instability. Bull Hosp Jt Dis Orthop Inst 1984;44(2):511.

Taleisnik J. Palmar carpal instability secondary to dislocation of the scaphoid and lunate: report of case and review of the literature. J Hand Surg [Am] 1982;7(6):606.

Taleisnik J. Post traumatic carpal instability. Clin Orthop 1980;149:73.

Taleisnik J. Triquetral hamate and triquetral lunate instabilities (medial carpal instability). Ann Chir Main 1984;3(4):331.

Taleisnik J. Ulnar variance in carpal instability. J Hand Surg [Am] 1987;12(2):205.

Vance RM, Gelberman RH, Evans EF. Scaphocapitate fractures: patterns of dislocation, mechanism of injury, and preliminary results of treatment. J Bone Joint Surg [Am] 1980;62(2):271.

Viegas SF, Patterson RM, Peterson PD, et al. Ulnar sided perilunate instability: an anatomic and biomechanical study. J Hand Surg [Am] 1990;15(2):268.

Viegas SF, Patterson RM, Peterson PD, et al. Evaluation of the biomechanical efficacy of limited intercarpal fusions for the treatment of scapholunate dissociation. J Hand Surg [Am] 1990;15(1):120.

Viegas SF, Tencer AF, Cantrell J, et al. Load transfer characteristics of the wrist. Part II. Perilunate instability. J Hand Surg [Am] 1987;12(6):978.

Weber ER. Concepts governing the rotational shift of the intercalated segment of the carpus. Orthop Clin North Am 1984;15(2):193.

10

Extrinsic Ligaments

*T*he extrinsic ligaments of the wrist maintain the longitudinal relationships of the forearm, carpal bones, and metacarpals. They are responsible for the proper articulation of the proximal row with the radius and triangular fibrocartilage (TFC), and of the distal carpal row with the proximal row. The extrinsic ligaments are primarily responsible for the stability of the distal radioulnar joint (DRUJ). They combine with the intrinsic ligaments and articular contours to limit normal rotational movements within the carpus and between the carpus and forearm. The hand will pronate and supinate to varying degrees within the carpus independent of the DRUJ. This motion is limited principally by the extrinsic ligaments, which also limit flexion and extension of the wrist. The integrity of the wrist in a coronal plane is maintained principally by the intrinsic ligaments.

Sprains of the extrinsic ligaments are common. Most wrist sprains require little treatment and will heal spontaneously if splinted sufficiently. Many sprains, however, are underdiagnosed. The extrinsic ligaments of the wrist may be stretched beyond their plastic limits, leaving segments of the carpus poorly supported and unstable. Ligaments can also be avulsed from their bony attachment, or can rupture completely in midsubstance.

Together, the extrinsic ligaments of the wrist comprise the thicker portion of the joint capsule. Where the capsule fibers course parallel to one another and have a distinct point of origin and insertion, they serve a common purpose and are referred to as specific ligaments. These ligaments are defined in detail in Chapter 5. However, the entire joint capsule is composed of linear fibers providing variable degrees of longitudinal and rotational support to the wrist between the discrete ligamentous structures. Any traction injury to the joint capsule technically should be considered a ligament sprain.

Severe sprains of the intrinsic ligaments cause longitudinal or rotational instability of the wrist, and can even allow dislocation of one or more carpal bones. The most commonly recognized and widely studied severe wrist sprains are those that cause lunate and perilunate dislocation. Other severe extrinsic ligament injuries also occur and may present with specific or subtle clinical signs. Many of these ligament injuries are not well understood. For example, the ligament injury or injuries that allow instability of the DRUJ have not been precisely defined. To choose the most advantageous position of immobilization following a slight to moderate wrist sprain, or to plan the ideal approach for ligament repair or reconstruction following severe sprains requires a good understanding of the anatomy of the extrinsic wrist ligaments and their respective functions.

On the volar side of the wrist, the extrinsic ligaments appear flat when examining and palpating the outer surface of the joint capsule. Internally, they stand in distinct relief. They can be examined well and palpated by means of arthroscopy in various joint positions. This is probably the most accurate means of examining extrinsic ligament injuries available.

The dorsal extrinsic ligaments are less well-defined. They also appear flat and barely distinguishable on examination of the outer surface of the capsule. During arthroscopic examination, they appear much less distinct than the volar ligaments, but sometimes can be recognized internally with the bright light and magnification provided by the arthroscope.

CLINICAL PRESENTATION

The extrinsic wrist ligaments provide longitudinal and rotational support; therefore, injuries result from excessive flexion, extension, and rotation. The examiner should attempt to elicit a precise description of the mechanism of injury. Swelling of the wrist may be generalized, but on close questioning patients can usually identify precisely the areas of maximal discomfort. Such questioning may be tedious, but is generally well worth the effort. Localized tenderness on palpation will further help to identify the injured extrinsic structures. Passively stretching specific ligaments helps to confirm the identification of the injured structures.

Radiographs should be taken in positions that stretch or stress suspected injured ligaments to look for subtle evidence of instability or widening of joint spaces in comparison with the uninjured side. Traction films may also be revealing.

Examining the wrist for rotational sprains can

be tricky. Pain on active pronation or supination usually implicates the DRUJ or the extensor carpi ulnaris (ECU) tendon. Aggravation of discomfort by ulnar deviation of the wrist suggests a torn TFC or possible ulnocarpal abutment.

Passive supination and pronation should be checked with the examiner holding first the hand, then the distal forearm (Fig. 10-1). Pain on passive pronation or supination delivered through the hand stresses the carpometacarpal (CMC), midcarpal, and radiocarpal intervals. Rotational stress applied by holding the distal forearm isolates the DRUJ. Hypersupination will add a volar translational force to the distal ulna; hyperpronation will add a dorsal translational force to the distal ulna. If there is pain with these motions, or if the ulna appears prominent, comparison should always be made with the uninjured side. A computed tomography (CT) scan of both wrists in full pronation and supination is most helpful in identifying instability of the DRUJ. If hemarthrosis is present, aspiration under fluoroscopic examination and injection of the wrist with 1% lidocaine (Xylocaine) will provide immediate pain relief and facilitate stress x-ray examination.

An important clue to avulsion or rupture of the volar or dorsal capsule is the presence of swelling in the volar or dorsal muscle compartments respectively. If tension or pain on palpation of the volar compartment is observed, each flexor tendon should be examined with the wrist in passive flexion to minimize pain from the volar capsule and isolate discomfort that may be caused by a flexor muscle or tendon injury. Similarly, if swelling or tenderness to palpation of the outcropping thenar muscles or extensor compartment is found, the extensors should be examined with the wrist held in passive extension to eliminate dorsal capsule pain and differentiate extensor muscle or tendon injury.

Without signs of carpal instability or ruptured joint capsule, sprains of extrinsic wrist ligaments should be treated with 3 to 6 weeks of splinting in a position that relaxes the injured ligament. In general, for the more commonly injured dorsal radiocarpal ligaments, the wrist should be placed in extension and radial deviation. For the dorsal ulnar ligaments, use extension and ulnar deviation (Fig. 10-2). If there is also evidence of ECU tendinitis or tenosynovitis, a clam shell splint or an above-elbow

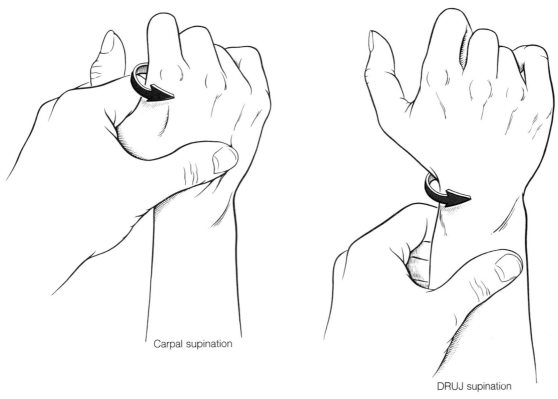

Carpal supination

DRUJ supination

FIGURE 10–1.
Passive supination can be applied through the patient's hand or forearm. Supinating or pronating the hand fully stresses the carpometacarpal, the midcarpal, and the radiocarpal intervals. Rotational force applied through the forearm stresses the distal radioulnar joint (DRUJ) and the triangular fibrocartilage complex.

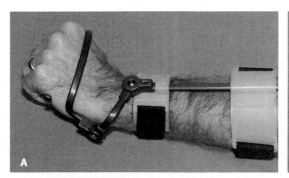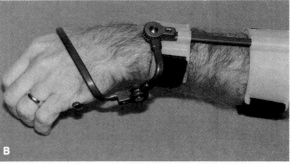

FIGURE 10–2.
A functional, limited-motion splint (Smith and Nephew DonJoy, Carlsbad, CA) is used to protect specific ligament injuries. The splint is pictured maintaining the wrist in (**A**) extension and radial deviation to protect dorsal radial ligaments, and (**B**) flexion and ulnar deviation to protect volar ulnar ligaments.

splint extension to maintain slight pronation is recommended to further eliminate stress on the ulnar side (Fig. 10-3).

Volar radiocarpal ligaments can be injured by hyperextension. Remember that the proximal carpal row rotates in the opposite direction of the hand in radial and ulnar deviation. Consequently, ligaments that insert on the proximal row are tight in radial deviation; the radioscaphocapitate (RSC) ligament is tight in ulnar deviation (Fig. 10-4). For sprains of the volar RSC ligament, immobilize the wrist in a position of flexion and radial deviation (Fig. 10-5). For the volar ulnocarpal ligaments that insert on the triquetrum and lunate, slight flexion with ulnar

deviation is appropriate. A functional, limited range splint will effectively protect specific ligaments while permitting some wrist mobility, a distinct advantage over cast immobilization (see Fig. 10-2).

Sprains of the supporting ligaments for the DRUJ can be difficult to manage. Opinions differ as to which structures stabilize this joint in pronation and in supination. Fortunately, when a sprain is present without discernible instability, the issue is less compelling than when reconstructive stabilizing procedures are required. In general, if a DRUJ sprain is more painful in forced pronation, immobilization in supination is appropriate. Conversely, if there is greater discomfort with passive supination of the forearm, splinting in pronation is advisable. A clam shell splint molded along the intermuscular septum of the forearm will prevent rotation in slender individuals. For larger extremities, an above-elbow splint is required to control rotation.

The positions discussed above will relax the respective ligaments when injured to allow healing in the most shortened position. Under no circumstances, however, should the wrist be immobilized in extreme positions.

ARTHROSCOPIC APPEARANCE

When injuries to the extrinsic ligaments of the wrist produce radiographic or clinical evidence of carpal instability, rupture of the capsule, or mechanical limitation of motion in the acute stage, arthroscopic examination of the wrist may be warranted. Arthroscopy will help identify any associated soft-tissue injury such as articular defects or rupture of the triangular fibrocartilage complex (TFCC), and to determine whether acute repair of the injured ligament may be advantageous. Similarly, when less severe sprains of the extrinsic ligaments fail to improve with appropriate immobilization, arthroscopic evaluation may be indicated to identify any associated occult pathology that might explain persistent symptoms.

There is a greater propensity for synovial hypertrophy on the dorsal aspect of the wrist joint than on the volar side. Acute injuries to the dorsal radiocarpal ligaments can be examined best from the 1-2 portal. The synovium covering the dorsal capsule will appear edematous, with increased vas-

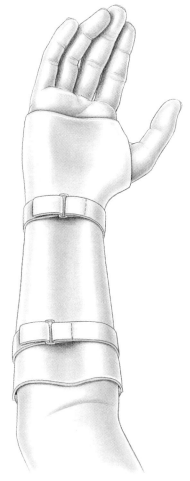

FIGURE 10–3.
A clam-shell splint molded between the radius and ulna will limit pronation and supination.

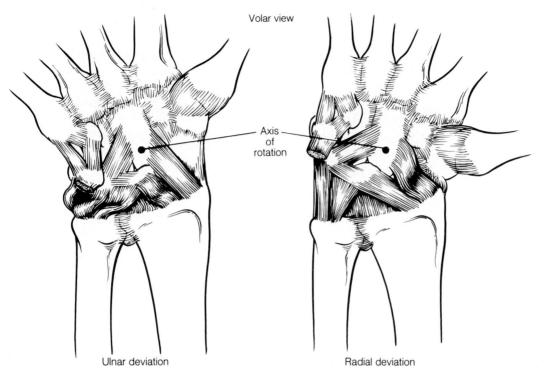

Volar view

Axis
of
rotation

Ulnar deviation   Radial deviation

FIGURE 10–4.

In ulnar and radial deviation, the center axis of rotation is through the capitate. In ulnar deviation, the radioscaphocapitate ligament is tight, and the radiolunate ligament is slack. In radial deviation, the converse is true.

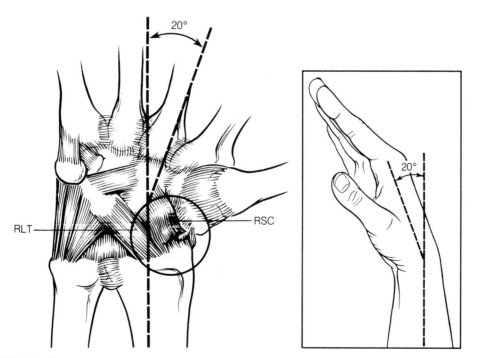

20°

RLT ——   —— RSC

20°

FIGURE 10–5.

For sprains of the volar radioscaphocapitate (RSC) ligament, immobilizing the wrist in flexion and radial deviation places this ligament in its most relaxed and protected position (*inset*). Except in the case of the volar radiolunotriquetral (RLT) ligament, sprains generally should be splinted with the hand deviated toward the site of maximal tenderness.

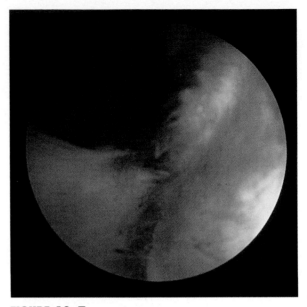

FIGURE 10–6.
Posttraumatic synovitis following hyperflexion injury with rupture of the dorsal radial capsule, as viewed from the 1-2 portal (right wrist).

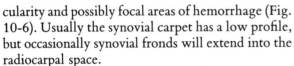

FIGURE 10–7.
An inflamed dorsal ulnar synovitis covering the floor of the extensor carpi ulnaris tendon sheath following traction injury. Viewed from the 3-4 portal (right wrist).

cularity and possibly focal areas of hemorrhage (Fig. 10-6). Usually the synovial carpet has a low profile, but occasionally synovial fronds will extend into the radiocarpal space.

On the ulnar side of the wrist, the most important dorsal ligamentous structure is actually the floor of the ECU tendon sheath. Injury to this structure is difficult to differentiate clinically from ECU tendinitis or subluxation, and the mechanism of injury for these conditions may be similar—usually flexion with extreme supination. When the dorsal ulnocarpal ligament is injured, hemorrhagic synovitis will be present along the dorsal ulnar capsule, extending to the articular disc of the TFCC and at times to the prestyloid recess (Fig. 10-7). There may also be a separation between the TFCC articular disc and the dorsal capsule (Fig. 10-8). Pronation and supination of the wrist and probing of the TFCC through the 6-U portal will help identify such injuries.

The dorsal extrinsic ligaments rarely rupture completely. They may, however, be avulsed from the radius, from the triquetrum or capitate, or from their narrow attachment along the dorsal rim of the proximal carpal row (Fig. 10-9). Avulsion of the dorsal capsule from its bony attachment to the radius can be seen best from the 1-2 or 3-4 portals. Ex-

tending the wrist, the arthroscope can be maneuvered over the dorsal rim of the radius to reveal exposed bone just proximal to the edge of the articular cartilage (Fig. 10-10). It may be necessary to retract the dorsal capsule with a probe from the ulnar side to identify this injury.

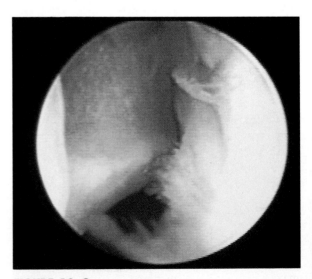

FIGURE 10–8.
Avulsion of the triangular fibrocartilage complex articular disc from the dorsal capsule, as viewed from 3-4 portal (right wrist).

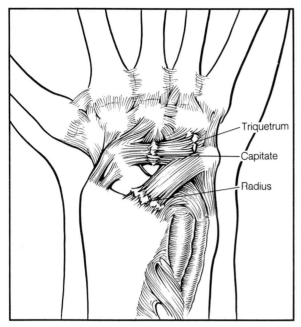

FIGURE 10–9.
Common sites of avulsion of the dorsal extrinsic ligaments are the radius, capitate, and triquetrum.

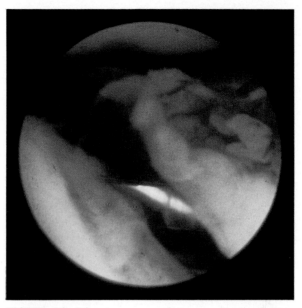

FIGURE 10–10.
Dorsal capsule avulsion with a small cartilage fragment from the dorsal rim of the radius, as viewed from the 1-2 portal (right wrist).

If the capsule is avulsed from the proximal carpal row, the arthroscope can be passed from the 3-4 portal into the midcarpal space. Follow the contour of the lunate or the dorsal aspect of the scaphoid distally. When the capsule is seen attaching to the waist of the scaphoid or to the distal dorsal rim of the lunate, follow that attachment across the dorsum of the wrist with the joint in extension. Hemorrhage and synovial hypertrophy is usually present but may be surprisingly minor. If any portion of the hamate, capitate, or the scaphotrapeziotrapezoid (STT) joint can be seen, the dorsal capsule has been avulsed.

Disruption of the capsule from its insertion on the distal carpal row is usually seen on the ulnar side of the wrist. From the radial midcarpal (RMC) portal, a large bare area on the capitate or hamate can be identified. Normally, the capsule attaches to these carpal bones along the margin of the articular cartilage, but may attach slightly more distal as a normal variant. The size of the exposed nonarticular surface of the capitate or hamate is therefore a critical consideration in the diagnosis of capsular avulsion and should take into account the precise location of maximal tenderness on physical examination. On rare occasions, the dorsal capsule may be stripped completely from its attachment on the distal carpal

row, permitting a view of the carpal metacarpal joints of the third, fourth, or fifth rays. This injury is rare, but should be investigated if clinical evaluation warrants.

On the volar side of the wrist, the extrinsic ligaments are readily identifiable. From radial to ulnar, beginning at the radial styloid, the RSC ligament and the broader radiolunotriquetral (RLT) ligament can be seen standing in relief against the volar capsule (Fig. 10-11). Behind the radial side of the synovial tuft, at the volar edge of the scapholunate intercarpal ligament, are the fibers of the flat radioscapholunate (RSL) ligament, also known as the ligament of Testut (Fig. 10-12). These ligaments can be seen from the 3-4 or the 1-2 portals. When injured, they may either stretch, rupture in midsubstance, or avulse from the radius. The overlying synovium will be swollen, boggy, and invariably hemorrhagic (Fig. 10-13). With severe injuries, capsule edema may obscure the cleavage planes between these ligaments. If only stretched, additional traction on the wrist will make the ligaments appear more distinct. However, if the volar ligaments have been avulsed from the radius, they will continue to appear boggy and lax despite increased traction. When any of these ligaments rupture in midsubstance, they tend to fold into the radiocarpal space

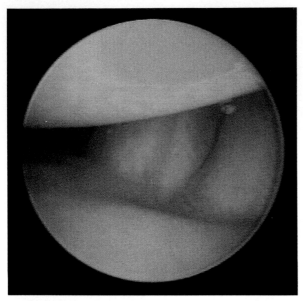

FIGURE 10—11.
Prominent volar radioscaphocapitate and radiolunotriquetral ligaments, as viewed from the 3-4 portal (right wrist).

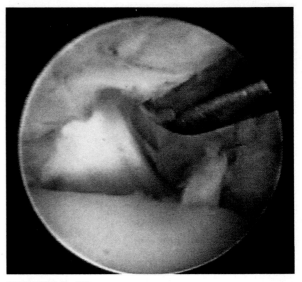

FIGURE 10—12.
A probe in the 4-5 portal retracts the volar synovial tuft to expose the radioscaphocapitate ligament of Testut. Viewed from the 3-4 portal (right wrist).

(Fig. 10-14). The invagination of ruptured fibers is reduced by wrist extension and additional traction, and is increased by wrist flexion or reduction of traction.

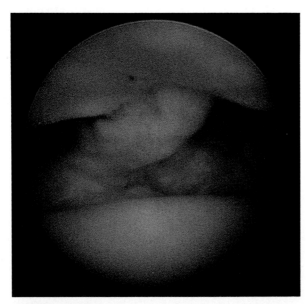

FIGURE 10—13.
Acute rupture of the volar radiolunotriquetral ligament. Note the edema, laxity, and acute hemorrhage in the ligament. Viewed from the 3-4 portal (right wrist).

Major sprains of the volar ulnocarpal ligaments have been observed only rarely. The ulnolunate and ulnotriquetral (UT) ligaments usually fail at their origin from the fossa of the ulnar head (Fig. 10-15). I have never observed a disruption of these ligaments distally.

Assessment of the integrity of the volar ulnocarpal ligaments requires palpation. The ligaments can be inspected most thoroughly with the arthroscope in the 6-U portal looking distally on the volar aspect of the triquetrum. A probe can be introduced through the 4-5 or 6-R portal to palpate the tension on these ligaments when the wrist is placed in extension and slight radial deviation. They never feel completely taut even when uninjured, but the lack of increased tension when the wrist is extended should raise suspicion of a significant stretch or avulsion injury.

Avulsion of the volar ulnocarpal ligaments from the ulna allows the TFCC articular disc to drift distally. With neutral or negative ulnar variance, an arthroscope can be introduced into the DRUJ proximal to the TFCC. The origin of the volar carpal ligaments cannot be readily identified, but avulsion of these ligaments will disclose in this area extreme proliferation of the volar synovium as a hemorrhagic amorphous mass. Blood is usually present in the DRUJ under these circumstances.

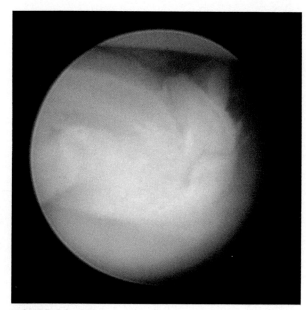

FIGURE 10–14.
A ruptured volar radiocarpal ligament folds into the radiocarpal space. Viewed from the 1-2 portal (right wrist).

TREATMENT

There is no apparent advantage to treating major injuries to the extrinsic ligaments of the wrist under arthroscopic control. Techniques for repairing or reattaching these ligaments have not yet been devised, and there is no place at present for reconstruction of wrist ligaments in the acute stages of injury. The advantage of arthroscopy in severe wrist sprains is to help define precisely which ligaments are involved and to what extent, and to discover the presence of other associated occult soft-tissue injuries that require treatment or that will affect the ultimate prognosis.

Commonly, major injuries to the extrinsic ligaments of the wrist are associated with disruption of the intrinsic intercarpal ligaments or the TFCC articular disc as well. Some of these injuries are best treated acutely to obtain optimal results. Arthroscopic treatment of intrinsic ligament injuries or certain tears of the TFC is possible and can often be

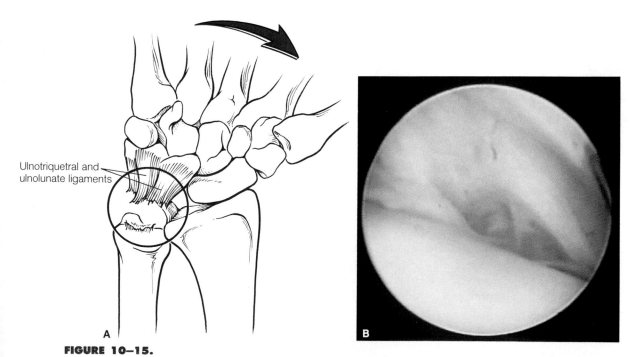

Ulnotriquetral and ulnolunate ligaments

FIGURE 10–15.
Extension and radial deviation injury rupturing the volar ulnocarpal ligaments proximal to the triangular fibrocartilage. (**A**) Volar representation. (**B**) The right wrist is seen in the distal radioulnar joint between the head of the ulna below and the proximal surface of the triangular fibrocartilage complex articular disc above. Note the frayed, edematous, slack ligaments.

accomplished at the time of arthroscopic evaluation of the extrinsic ligament injury.

After establishing a diagnosis of specific ligament injuries and any associated lesions, the initial treatment approach to the extrinsic ligament is usually nonoperative. This is predicated on the fact that the hand and wrist have an abundant blood supply and are especially prone to posttraumatic fibrosis. Using this tendency to advantage, appropriate splinting and controlled mobilization avoiding stress to the injured structures will usually result in scarring of the ligament and adequate restoration of function and stability.

If irregular shards of synovium, fibrin clots, or loose tags of ligament are present, they should be shaved from the joint at the time of the arthroscopic examination. The wrist is then immobilized in an appropriate position to relax the injured ligament as described above. All uninjured joints of the hand are mobilized immediately. After 2 weeks, the wrist also is mobilized passively through ranges that place no additional stress or tension on the injured ligament. Early mobilization reduces adhesion formation, facilitates articular cartilage nutrition, and mitigates unwanted fibrosis of uninjured capsular structures.

Splinting of severe sprains should be continued for 6 to 12 weeks depending on the degree of injury, the patient's general joint laxity, and the density of his connective tissue, which is thought to be an index of potential for scar formation. Functional splinting is then recommended for an additional 2 months or more to protect against extremes of motion that would stretch the healing ligament.

The two exceptions to this conservative treatment approach are cases in which a specific ligament or ligaments are avulsed cleanly from bone, or in which there is apparent carpal instability. Ligament or capsule avulsion is best treated in the acute stage by direct primary reattachment. This can be accomplished with staples, suture anchors, or sutures through drill holes in bone (Fig. 10-16). Clean avulsions of capsule or extrinsic ligaments provide an opportunity for anatomic repair with an excellent prognosis.

When extrinsic ligament injuries produce obvious carpal instability, a difficult judgment must be made. Some cases are best treated with immediate open reduction, pin fixation, and ligament repair;

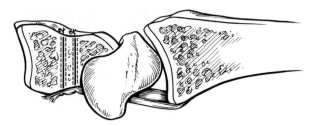

FIGURE 10–16.
Procedure for acute repair of a ruptured volar radioscaphocapitate ligament. Sutures through the ligament are passed through drill holes in the capitate and tied dorsally.

others are treated best with closed reduction, percutaneous pinning, and immobilization in an appropriate position as described above. Remember that extrinsic ligaments are all flat and indistinct when viewed from the outside surface of the joint capsule. Further obscured by tearing and hemorrhage, these ligaments may be difficult if not impossible to identify and repair with appropriate tension. Surgical trauma can compound the initial injury, and remaining ligaments can be disrupted in the course of surgical exposure. Depending on the degree of apparent soft-tissue injury and the surgeon's comfort with soft-tissue wrist surgery, it may be preferable to accurately reduce the carpal bones with pin fixation and allow scar formation to reconstitute a collagen mass. The collagen mass subsequently can be used for a staged capsulorrhaphy or ligamentoplasty.

PREFERRED TREATMENT

In general, extrinsic ligament injuries of the wrist fall into one of four categories:

1. Slight to moderate sprains without disruptions of the carpus
2. Severe sprains with rupture of the capsule, but without disruption of the carpus
3. Ligament avulsion without carpal dissociation
4. Acute carpal instability.

Patients who present with a history of bending or twisting trauma to the wrist, localized tenderness and swelling, but with soft forearm muscle compartments and normal stress x-rays, are splinted in an appropriate position for relaxation of the involved ligament for 3 to 6 weeks. This group is considered to have a mild to moderate wrist sprain without capsule disruption.

Patients who have a similar history but with swelling or tension in the distal forearm or with radiographic evidence of carpal dissociation are considered for early arthroscopic examination under general or regional anesthesia. An inflow catheter is placed in the 6-U portal, and the arthroscope is introduced initially through the 3-4 portal for inspection of the volar ligaments, the TFCC, the proximal row intrinsic ligaments, and the articular surfaces. If the physical examination suggests a dorsal capsule injury, the arthroscope is then reintroduced through the 1-2 portal for inspection of the dorsal ligaments. If an injury to the volar ulnocarpal ligaments is suspected, the second arthroscopic entry is through the 6-U portal with inflow on the arthroscope sheath.

Patients with midsubstance ruptures of extrinsic ligaments or a capsule with no radiographic evidence of carpal dissociation, and in whom no other intraarticular pathology is found at arthroscopy, are treated with cast immobilization in an appropriate position to relax the injured ligaments for 2 weeks. Thereafter a splint is applied and limited mobilization is provided for an additional 4 to 10 weeks. A functional brace is used to block extremes of stressful motion for 2 to 4 months, depending on the severity of injury.

Patients who have distinct ligament or capsule avulsion at the time of arthroscopy, but who have no other intraarticular pathology and no radiographic evidence of carpal instability are candidates for primary capsulorrhaphy or ligamentoplasty. The precise location of the ligament avulsion is identified with marker needles introduced under arthroscopic control. An incision is then planned to provide direct access to the involved ligament with as little dissection as possible. The site of bone attachment is freshened with a small curette or burr. Pneumatically driven staples (3-M, Minneapolis, MN) or suture anchors (Mitek Surgical Products, Inc., Norwood, MA) are used to reattach the ligament or capsule. The staples and anchors are preferred because they obviate the need for drill holes that may corticalize or possibly compromise carpal circulation. They also obviate the need for counter incisions to retrieve and tie sutures and for pull-out wires that can pro-

vide an avenue for bacterial ingress. A cast is applied for 2 weeks, after which treatment is the same as described for midsubstance capsule or ligament ruptures.

When stress or traction radiographs indicate unusual widening of intercarpal spaces or subluxation within the carpus compared with the opposite normal wrist, arthroscopic examination is performed early as described above, preferably within 2 weeks of injury. Usually an associated tear of one or more intrinsic carpal ligaments or the TFCC will be seen. These injuries are treated acutely (see Chaps. 8 and 9). Hemarthrosis and other debris are cleared from the joint. The carpal bones are reduced anatomically with a combination of arthroscopic and radiographic control, and are pinned in place with .035- or .045-inch wires crossing as few articular surfaces as possible. Avulsion injuries of extrinsic ligaments are treated as described above by staple or suture anchor reattachment. The wrist is placed in an appropriate position to relax the injured extrinsic ligaments, and is immobilized in a long-arm cast for 3 weeks (for 6 weeks if the DRUJ is involved). A short-arm cast is then applied for 6 additional weeks. The cast is removed or windowed over pin tracks for inspection and aseptic cleansing every 2 weeks. The pins are removed after approximately 8 weeks. Gradual mobilization is then allowed over a period of 4 weeks, and a functional brace is applied for 2 more months.

These regimens may vary slightly depending on the patient's general joint laxity and connective tissue density. They have proven to be reliable techniques for maintaining carpal stability with minimal surgical trauma, reasonably early return to function, and few complications.

BIBLIOGRAPHY

Bartosh RA, Saldana MJ. Intraarticular fractures of the distal radius: a cadaveric study to determine if ligamentotaxis restores radiopalmar tilt. J Hand Surg [Am] 1990;15(1):18.

Blatt G. Capsulodesis and reconstructive hand surgery: capsulodesis following excision of the distal ulna. Hand Clin 1987;3(1):81.

Carroll RE, Coyle MP Jr. Dysfunction of the pisotriquetral joint: treatment by excision of the pisiform. J Hand Surg [Am] 1985;10(5):703.

Drewniany JJ, Palmer AK, Flatt AE. The scaphotrapezial

ligament complex: an anatomic and biomechanical study. J Hand Surg [Am] 1985;10(4):492.

Drewniany JJ, Palmer AK. Injuries to the distal radioulnar joint. Orthop Clin North Am 1986;17(3):451.

Fayman M, Hugo B, deWet H. Simultaneous dislocation of all five carpal metacarpal joints. Plast Reconstr Surg 1988;82(1):151.

Frykman E. Dislocations of the triquetrum: case report. Scand J Plast Reconstr Surg 1980;14(2):205.

Garcia-Elias M, Au KN, Cooney WP III, Linscheid RL, Chao EY. Stability of the transverse carpal arch: an experimental study. J Hand Surg [Am] 1989;14(2):277.

Garcia-Elias M, Dobyns JH, Cooney WP III, Linscheid RL. Traumatic axial dislocations of the carpus. J Hand Surg [Am] 1989;14(3):446.

Hastings DE, Silver RL. Intercarpal arthrodesis in the management of chronic carpal instability after trauma. J Hand Surg [Am] 1984;9(6):834.

Jasmine MS, Packer JW, Edwards GS Jr. Irreducible transcaphoid perilunate dislocation. J Hand Surg [Am] 1988;13(2):212.

King GJ, McMurtry RY, Rubenstein JD, Ogston NG. Computerized tomography of the distal radioulnar joint: correlation with ligamentous pathology in a cadaveric model. J Hand Surg [Am] 1986;11(5):711.

Logan SE, Nowak MD. Intrinsic and extrinsic wrist ligaments: biomechanical and functional differences. ISA Trans 1988;27(3):37.

Mino DE, Palmer AK, Levinsohn EM. Radiography and computerized tomography in the diagnosis of incongruity of the distal radioulnar joint: a prospective study. J Bone Joint Surg [Am] 1985;67(2):247.

Mino DE, Palmer AK, Levinsohn EM. The role of radiography and computerized tomography in the diagnosis of subluxation and dislocation of the distal radioulnar joint. J Hand Surg [Am] 1983;8(1):23.

Paley D, Rubenstein JD, McMurtry RY. Irreducible dislocation of distal radioulnar joint. Orthop Rev 1986;15(4):228.

Scheffler R, Armstrong D, Hutton L. Computed tomographic diagnosis of distal radioulnar joint disruption. J Can Assoc Radiol 1984;35(2):212.

Siegert JJ, Frassica FJ, Amadio PC. Treatment of chronic perilunate dislocations. J Hand Surg [Am] 1988;13(2):206.

Space TC, Louis DS, Francis I, Braunstein EM. CT findings in distal radioulnar dislocations. J Comput Assist Tomogr 1986;10(4):689.

Taleisnik J. Post traumatic ulnar translation of the carpus. J Hand Surg [Am] 1987;12(2):180.

Vance RM, Gelberman RH, Evans EF. Scaphocapitate fractures: patterns of dislocation, mechanisms of injury and preliminary results of treatment. J Bone Joint Surg [Am] 1980;62(2):271.

Viegas SF. Intraarticular ganglion of the dorsal interosseous scapholunate ligament: a case for arthroscopy. Arthroscopy 1986;2(2):93.

Volz RG, Lieb M, Benjamin J. Biomechanics of the wrist. Clin Orthop 1980;149:112.

Watson HK, Black DM. Instabilities of the wrist. Hand Clin 1987;3(1):103.

Weber ER. Concepts governing the rotational shift of the intercalated segment of the carpus. Orthop Clin North Am 1984;15(2):193.

Wechsler RJ, Wehbe MA, Rifkin MD, Edeiken J, Branch HM. Computed tomography diagnosis of distal radioulnar subluxation. Skeletal Radiol 1987;16(1):1.

Youm Y, Flatt AE. Kinematics of the wrist. Clin Orthop 1980;149:21.

11

Intraarticular Fractures
of the Distal Radius and Carpals

FRACTURES OF THE RADIUS

Nonarticular fractures of the distal radius occur frequently and in all age groups. Any angulation or shortening deformation of the radius will affect the distal radioulnar joint (DRUJ) and may tear the triangular fibrocartilage complex (TFCC; Fig. 11-1). This is the primary reason that accurate reduction of the fracture and restoration of length to the radius is desirable. Fracture planes in the distal radius often disrupt the articular surface. Although in many cases patients seem to achieve satisfactory wrist function despite incomplete fracture reduction, ideal long-term function requires optimal reduction of the fracture and restoration of normal anatomic form.

The primary tenet of articular fracture care in all joints, large and small, is accurate reconstruction of the articular surface. In the wrist, however, depressed central fracture fragments and many peripheral fragments cannot be reduced by closed manipulation and capsular traction. Conventional techniques for open reduction and stabilization of these fragments introduce additional surgical trauma. Important capsular and ligamentous structures about the wrist must be incised or released to gain access to the articular surface. There is then the dilemma between immobilization for soft-tissue healing and early motion to stimulate articular cartilage and to prevent adhesions and arthrosis.

Based on the advantages and excellent results of reducing and stabilizing tibial plateau fractures under arthroscopic control, similar techniques have been developed for articular fractures of the distal radius. Arthroscopic reduction and internal fixation (ARIF) of radius fractures causes minimal surgical trauma and provides good visualization of the joint surface for accurate reassembly of articular fracture fragments. Soft-tissue healing considerations are negligible if there has been no ligament injury from the original trauma. Injured ligaments or cartilage are more likely to be recognized with an early arthroscopic examination than with clinical and x-ray evaluation alone.

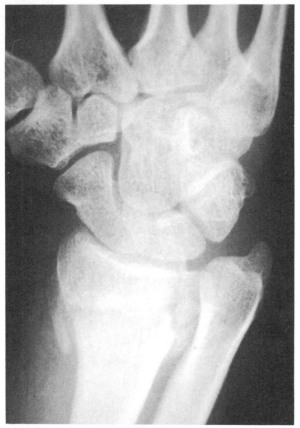

FIGURE 11–1.
Radiograph of comminuted impacted distal radius fracture with shortening and disruption of the distal radioulnar joint.

Clinical Presentation

The presenting symptoms and signs of distal radius fractures are well-known. A conventional series of radiographs is the most important means of assessing fracture comminution and fracture displacement. If there is any apparent disruption of the articular surface of the radius after closed manipulative reduction of the fracture, computed tomography (CT) evaluation should be considered. Computed tomography is the best noninvasive means of assessing the number and displacement of articular fragments (see Fig. 2-31). If fracture lines on the articular surface are not narrow and uniform, if cortical fragments at the edge of the joint surface are angulated, or if the sagittal and coronal measurements of the distal radius are enlarged compared with the opposite side, im-

proved reduction under arthroscopic control is indicated.

Arthroscopic Appearance

The ideal time to perform arthroscopic reduction of distal radius fractures is 2 to 4 days after injury. Earlier attempts are likely to encounter too much bleeding from the fracture surfaces; later attempts will find excessive fibrin precipitate in the joint from the hemarthrosis. This fibrin may be tedious to remove.

There is always more fracture debris in the joint than plain radiographs reveal. Blood, cartilage fragments, and bone crumbs are usually present. Fracture lines are readily apparent, and some fragment surfaces may be depressed or impacted.

Radial styloid fracture lines (chauffeur) run from anterior to posterior across the scaphoid facet. Die-punch fractures will usually have similar sagittal fracture lines across the scaphoid facet, with a second fracture line or more in the coronal plane originating at the sigmoid notch and crossing the lunate facet to join the first fracture line (Fig. 11-2). The dorsal ulnar and volar ulnar fragments will vary in size, but usually the dorsal ulnar fragment is smaller and may be depressed. Either of these primary fragments might be further comminuted. Blood will cling to areas of damaged articular cartilage. Torn or stretched ligaments will also appear blood stained and edematous. The TFCC is likely to be torn

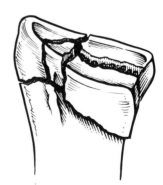

FIGURE 11–2.
Comminuted intraarticular distal radius fracture. Typical die-punch configuration with depressed impacted dorsal ulnar fragment. Notice the disruption of the distal radioulnar joint as well as the radiocarpal articulation.

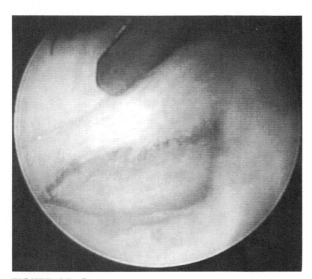

FIGURE 11–3.

An incidental tear in the triangular fibrocartilage complex (TFCC) secondary to distal radius fracture. Note the prominent ulnar head seen through the TFCC tear secondary to radial shortening. Viewed through the 3-4 portal (right wrist).

and should be explored thoroughly with a probe (Fig. 11-3).

Treatment

Initially, an attempt should be made to reduce the fracture by closed manipulation under anesthesia, with care not to traumatize the median nerve or ecchymotic skin. On arthroscopic examination, the radiocarpal space will be filled with blood and clot. This space must first be cleansed, a process that can be tedious and lengthy. A power shaver operated at medium speed is the most effective instrument for this task. A small soft-bristle brush is also helpful to spool up a tenacious clot and help remove it. Each fracture line should be as clean as possible so that no occult fracture planes are missed and fracture reduction can be monitored accurately. Bone crumbs can be removed with a small grasping forceps.

When the joint is clean, the mobility of each displaced fragment should be tested by pressing the articular surfaces or cortical edges with a small dissector. This will usually express more blood from the fracture planes, which can be cleared simply by continuous irrigation. Depressed and displaced fragments can be mobilized by inserting the dissector

into the fracture lines and prying them apart gently. Some fracture fragments may be nondisplaced with no separation of the fracture lines. These fragment relationships should not be disturbed.

Reduction of the fracture begins with the largest articular fragment—usually the volar ulnar fragment—to which each successively smaller fragment is assembled and pinned (Fig. 11-4). In this way, minor imperfections in reduction should involve only the smallest fragments. A smooth, small-diameter K-wire 3 to 4 inches long is drilled into the midportion of each fragment parallel to the articular surface, avoiding extensor tendons and the radial artery. If a fragment is depressed, two pins may be necessary to allow leverage without rotation of the fragment. Using the pins as handles, each fragment can be elevated and maneuvered into anatomic position. After all fragments are elevated to restore normal joint contour, the fracture lines are closed by applying external pressure at the base of each pin. When the fracture gaps are closed, the pins are advanced into adjacent fragments. It is unnecessary for the pins to cross fracture lines perpendicularly.

Occasionally, fracture lines will spring open despite pin fixation. This is most likely to occur in very hard or very soft bone. In hard bone, deeper cancellous surfaces may not be perfectly matched, even when the articular fracture line is completely reduced and closed. More compression is required to overcome this mismatch of cancellous surfaces than can be obtained with a single pin. In soft osteoporotic bone, a single smooth pin may not have enough distal purchase to stabilize the fracture.

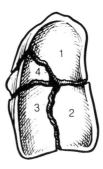

FIGURE 11–4.

Comminuted articular fracture of the radius. Numbers represent the order in which fragments should be reduced to one another, beginning with the largest articular fragment and progressing to the smallest.

In such cases, a second pin crossing the first at a 60° to 90° angle may add sufficient stability. Even better purchase and more compression can be obtained in such cases by inserting a cannulated Herbert–Whipple intraosseous screw (Zimmer, Warsaw, IN) over the first wire (Fig. 11-5). Inserted through a 5- to 6-mm incision, the screw provides secure purchase of adjacent fragments and achieves gentle compression through differing thread pitch at opposite ends of the screw. It can be buried completely within the bone and left permanently. When all fragments have been reduced and stabilized, an intraoperative radiograph should determine minor adjustments of the depth of the pins. Each pin is then bent and cut short.

Bone grafting is unnecessary even after depressed fragments have been reduced. The pins just beneath the subchondral bone provide excellent fragment stability. Metaphyseal voids fill readily with cancellous bone.

Additional fixation may be necessary in three specific circumstances. First, after reconstitution of the articular surface, the palmar tilt of the epiphysis should be restored by manipulation. In the interest of early motion, it may sometimes be necessary to add an additional pin from the radial styloid to the opposite metaphyseal cortex to maintain palmar tilt. Second, if there has been severe impaction of fragments and shortening of the radius or excessive comminution of the metaphysis of the radius, an external fixator should be considered to maintain length (Fig. 11-6). Finally, Smith's fractures are inherently unstable and nearly always require application of a volar buttress plate. It is easier to apply the plate after arthroscopic reduction and pin fixation of the articular surface.

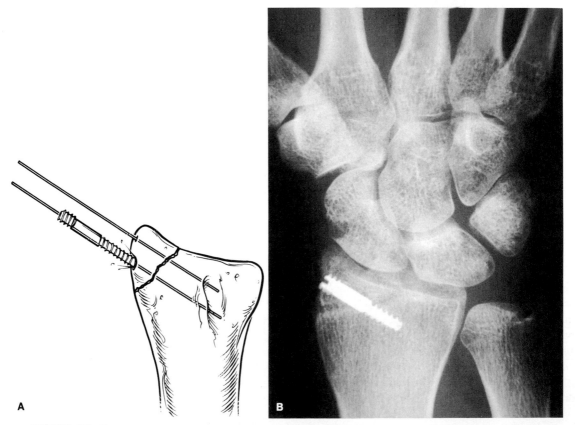

FIGURE 11–5.

A cannulated Herbert–Whipple screw can be used to provide additional compression of fracture fragments when the reduction remains springy and tends to gap open over smooth K-wires. (**A**) Insertion technique. (**B**) Two weeks after fixation the secondary K-wire is removed. The Herbert–Whipple intraosseous screw is buried beneath the cortex, causing no irritation. Variably pitched threads secure fracture reduction.

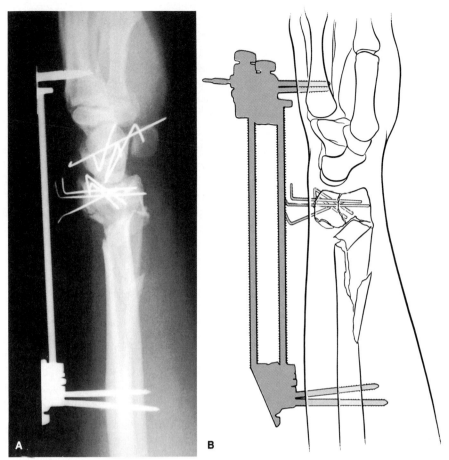

FIGURE 11–6.
Severely comminuted distal radius fracture involving metaphysis and articular surface. Following arthroscopic reduction and internal fixation of the articular fragments, the epiphysis is reduced to the diaphysis, and length is maintained with an external fixator. Fixators are used only when there is loss of cortical bone support in the metaphysis.

Postoperative management should strive for early mobilization of the wrist. A volar splint applied for 7 to 10 days can be removed thereafter by reliable patients for brief periods of active motion. Unreliable patients should be placed in a cast. The elbow need not be immobilized unless there is an associated ulna fracture or the stability of the DRUJ has been compromised.

Preferred Method

The forearm is prepped and sterilely draped, and a compressive elastic bandage or Coban (3M, Minneapolis, MN) is wrapped about the forearm to retard fluid extravasation into muscle compartments through the fracture planes. With 10 to 15 pounds of traction applied to the index and long fingers, a closed manipulative reduction is attempted. The Traction Tower is then adjusted into flexion or extension as the fracture alignment requires. Extensor tendons and the radial artery are marked with a skin pen, and portals are identified. With an inflow cannula in the 6-U portal, the arthroscope is placed in the 3-4 portal, and the joint is lavaged thoroughly. A 4-5 portal is established to remove clots, fibrin, cartilage debris, and bone crumbs.

When all fracture lines can be seen, fragments are disimpacted with a dissector by prying between fracture lines. Selecting a location near the midportion of each fragment and between marked tendons, a 25-gauge needle is inserted through the capsule.

The needle is directed over the fragment, across the fracture line, and toward a larger adjacent fragment. This needle is a direction guide for the insertion of K-wires. Drill a .045-inch K-wire percutaneously into the fracture fragment 6 to 8 mm proximal to the guide needle, in the direction of the needle and parallel to the joint surface. Remove the needle, and manipulate the fragment into its normal position. Each fragment is likewise reduced, beginning with the larger fragments and proceeding sequentially to the smaller ones. The fracture lines are compressed to close them, and the pins are advanced into the respective adjacent fragments. It may be possible to transfix three or more fragments with a single pin.

A radiograph in two planes confirms proper reduction and pin position (Fig. 11-7). A cannulated Herbert–Whipple screw is inserted if the fracture lines tend to spread. The palmar tilt is restored, and any required additional fixation to the radial shaft is applied. In most cases the extremity can be left in the Traction Tower for the application of ancillary fixation.

The pins are bent and cut short. They are wrapped with Xeroform gauze, and bandages are applied to incorporate a volar plaster splint or cast as described earlier. Pins are removed without anesthesia 3 to 6 weeks postoperatively depending on the degree of comminution and bone density.

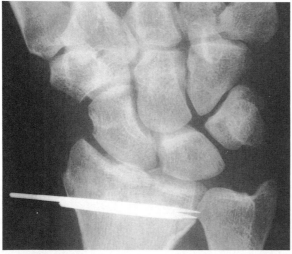

FIGURE 11–7.
An intraoperative radiograph confirms satisfactory reduction and pin placement following arthroscopic reduction and internal fixation.

Clinical Results

Treating articular fractures of the radius with ARIF has proven remarkably successful in restoring articular contours, achieving union, and preventing joint stiffness from fracture immobilization (Fig. 11-8). Patients seem to have less fracture pain after stabilization of the fragments. They appreciate the reduced period of confinement and are generally compliant with mobilization instructions.

We have seen no instance of reflex sympathetic dystrophy or nonunion. Reduction was lost 2 to 3 weeks postoperatively in one osteoporotic patient with a Smith's fracture in whom a buttress plate was not applied. A farmer with a severely comminuted epiphyseal and metaphyseal fracture treated with ARIF and an ancillary external fixator suffered a spontaneous rupture of the extensor pollicis longus (EPL) at Lister's tubercle 2 years later. He has achieved full function after tenorrhaphy but lacks complete thumb flexion. A third patient, steroid-dependent with systemic lupus erythematosus and bilateral intraarticular radius fractures, has had slightly worse stiffness in her metacarpophalangeal and intraphalangeal joints since injury, but this is not thought to be a function of her treatment.

FRACTURES OF THE SCAPHOID

Fractures of the scaphoid can be difficult treatment problems. It has been stated that 90% of scaphoid fractures will eventually heal if immobilized long enough. Unfortunately, the union may be deformed and immobilization may entail an above elbow thumb spica cast and still allow motion. The duration of casting may be 6 months or more. Few patients can tolerate those requirements today, emotionally or economically. In addition, the consequences of immobilizing an extremity for prolonged periods are deleterious and unacceptable.

If there is a better means of reducing deformity, hastening healing, and reducing immobilization with an acceptable level of risk, it is overdue. Clinical identification of scaphoid fractures prone to delayed union, nonunion, or malunion remains imprecise.

Herbert has proposed that all displaced fractures be treated with open reduction and internal fixation.[1] However, essentially nondisplaced fractures (slight

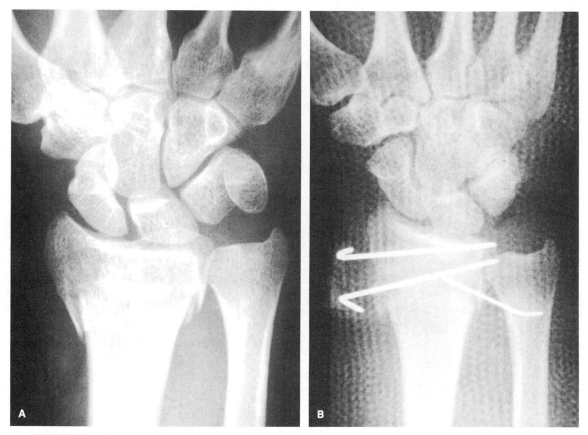

FIGURE 11–8.
(**A**) Three-part intraarticular distal radius fracture with shortening. (**B**) Status after arthroscopic reduction and internal fixation. Note the restoration of radius length and articular contour.

translation or minimal angulation) may also develop delayed union or nonunion, and can angulate secondarily during cast immobilization. Fractures most likely to heal uneventfully with casting often require 12 to 16 weeks of job modification, lost time from work, or withdrawal from an entire sports season. For these reasons, alternative treatment measures have been sought to provide equal or better results with less risk, less economic consequence, and with greater convenience to the patient.

Nonunion of a scaphoid fracture is occasionally well-tolerated, sometimes even not noticed. However, even these patients usually develop symptomatic arthrosis of the wrist eventually. The characteristic pattern of degeneration has been thoroughly documented. Humpback deformity occurs with flexion of the distal fragment and dorsal angulation at the fracture site (Fig. 11-9). Articular changes

and subchondral sclerosis occur first at the radioscaphoid interval (Fig. 11-10). Osteophytes may cause elongation of the radial styloid. Degenerative loss of articular surface progresses rapidly to the capitolunate interval. Treatment of the nonunion should be instituted if possible before degenerative changes occur. Most common approaches involve reduction of the deformity and bone grafting, with or without internal fixation.

Herbert–Whipple Screw Fixation

The development of the Herbert–Whipple intraosseous fixation screw and its unique application device (Zimmer, Warsaw, IN) allows essentially nondisplaced scaphoid fractures to be compressed and stabilized internally with minimally invasive surgical

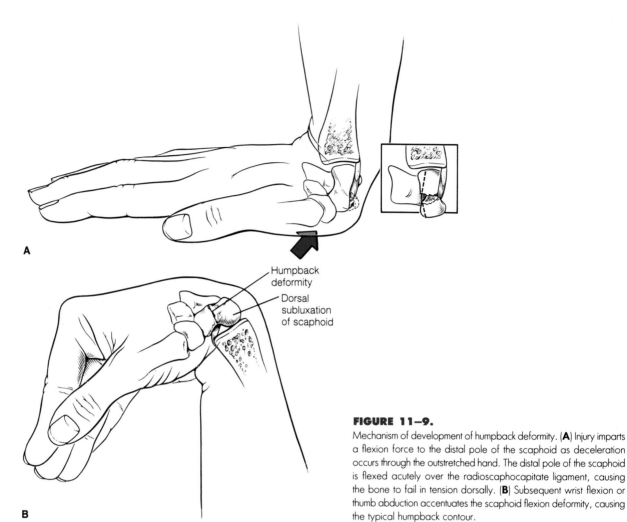

A

Humpback
deformity

Dorsal
subluxation
of scaphoid

B

FIGURE 11–9.
Mechanism of development of humpback deformity. (**A**) Injury imparts
a flexion force to the distal pole of the scaphoid as deceleration
occurs through the outstretched hand. The distal pole of the scaphoid
is flexed acutely over the radioscaphocapitate ligament, causing
the bone to fail in tension dorsally. (**B**) Subsequent wrist flexion or
thumb abduction accentuates the scaphoid flexion deformity, causing
the typical humpback contour.

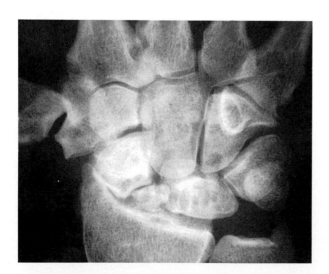

FIGURE 11–10.
Radiograph of typical advanced degenerative pattern following scaphoid nonunion. Note the elongation of the radial styloid, the sclerosis
and articular cartilage loss between the styloid and scaphoid distal
pole, and the increased sclerosis at the capitolunate articulation.

techniques and with arthroscopic assistance. The surgical risk and sequelae are therefore small. External casting can be drastically reduced, if not eliminated.

This primary surgical approach to nondisplaced and minimally displaced scaphoid fractures is in many ways more conservative than prolonged cast immobilization. It minimizes stiffness, atrophy, and cartilage deterioration, and allows better hygiene than casting. It requires less activity modification and permits an earlier return to productivity for those who work with their hands, thereby reducing the economic cost of the injury. In addition, internal fixation reduces the chance of delayed angulation of the fracture.

The device also can be used for internal fixation of scaphoid nonunions after open reduction and bone grafting (Fig. 11-11). However, its arthroscopic uses are only suitable for essentially nondisplaced or completely reducible fractures of the scaphoid.

Arthroscopic Appearance

Fractures of the scaphoid may enter the radiocarpal space, but they always involve the midcarpal space (Fig. 11-12). Hemarthrosis may be copious or slight. The fracture line usually has minimal gap and is seen best along the concave surface of the scaphoid

in the midcarpal space. Fibrin or clot fragments extrude from the fracture line. The scapholunate ligament is rarely injured in association with a scaphoid fracture.

Treatment

Displaced or angulated fractures of the scaphoid should be treated primarily with open reduction and internal fixation. Nondisplaced fractures in patients who can commit to several weeks of cast immobilization are best treated with a long-arm thumb spica cast. Consideration should be given to incorporating the index and long fingers in an intrinsic plus position to assure absolute immobilization. Patients with nondisplaced fractures who cannot commit to

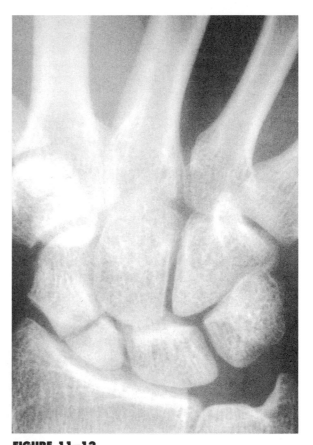

FIGURE 11-12.
Minimally displaced low-waist fracture of the scaphoid. The fracture line enters both the radiocarpal and midcarpal spaces. This fracture pattern is ideal for arthroscopically assisted internal fixation.

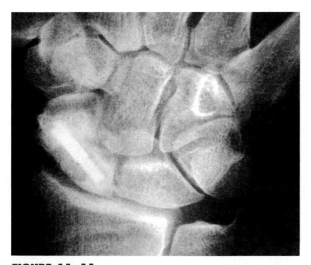

FIGURE 11-11.
Herbert–Whipple screw fixation of scaphoid nonunion with cortical cancellous bone graft shown 4 weeks postoperatively.

prolonged casting or those with essentially nondisplaced fractures of the scaphoid are candidates for ARIF.

Preferred Method

Only the arthroscopically assisted treatment technique will be described here. After gentle prepping and draping to avoid displacement of the fracture, a 12- to 15-mm incision is made centered over the volar tubercle of the trapezium just radial to the flexor carpi radialis tendon (Fig. 11-13*A*). The scaphotrapezial joint is identified and opened through a transverse capsulotomy. A T-shaped incision is made in the capsule and periosteum over the trapezium, meeting the transverse capsulotomy

(Fig. 11-13*B*). Capsular flaps are turned distally by subperiosteal dissection.

The scaphoid tubercle is then excised with a $^3/_{16}$-inch osteotome (Fig. 11-13*C*). Enough of the tubercle should be removed to expose a portion of the distal articular surface of the scaphoid where the screw will be introduced.

The forearm is then positioned vertically in the Traction Tower with 10 pounds of axial traction applied to the index and long fingers. The arthroscope is introduced very gently through the radial midcarpal (RMC) portal. To avoid applying excessive pressure during insertion of the arthroscope sheath and trocar, spread the subcutaneous tissue and lance the capsule with a No. 11 scalpel. After introducing the arthroscope sheath, the joint is flushed briefly. An inflow cannula is inserted in the ulnar

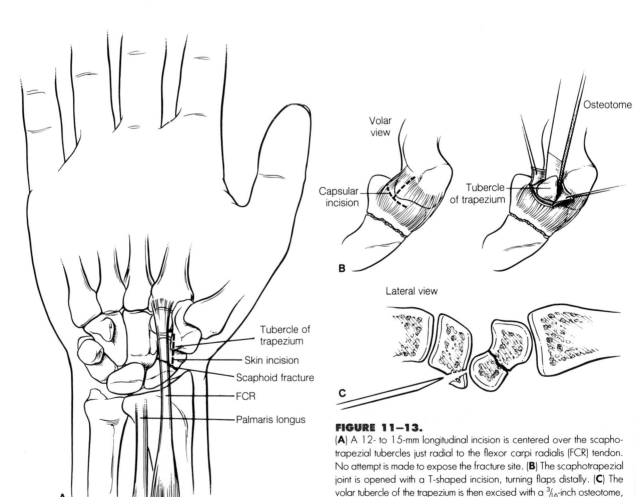

Tubercle of trapezium

Skin incision

Scaphoid fracture

FCR

Palmaris longus

Volar view

Capsular incision

Osteotome

Tubercle of trapezium

Lateral view

FIGURE 11—13.

(**A**) A 12- to 15-mm longitudinal incision is centered over the scapho-trapezial tubercles just radial to the flexor carpi radialis (FCR) tendon. No attempt is made to expose the fracture site. (**B**) The scaphotrapezial joint is opened with a T-shaped incision, turning flaps distally. (**C**) The volar tubercle of the trapezium is then excised with a $^3/_{16}$-inch osteotome, exposing the distal articular surface of the scaphoid.

midcarpal (UMC) portal, out of the way of fracture instrumentation. The hemarthrosis is then cleared completely, and the fracture line is examined for any evidence of displacement or angulation.

Small degrees of angulation or displacement can usually be reduced by placing the wrist in extension or supination, thereby reversing the humpback deformity and closing fracture lines. If this maneuver is unsuccessful, .045-inch K-wires can be inserted percutaneously into the scaphoid tubercle volarly and into the proximal pole dorsally to manipulate the fracture fragments. Anatomic reduction should be confirmed by radiograph or C-arm fluoroscopy.

The arthroscope is transferred to the 3-4 portal, and the inflow cannula is moved to the arthroscopy sheath or the 6-U portal. A 1-2 portal is established and dilated to admit the target hook of the compression jig. The jig should be maneuvered in the radiocarpal space under direct vision along the proximal pole of the scaphoid to a point approximately 1 mm from the scapholunate ligament along the proximal dorsal contour of the scaphoid articular surface (Fig. 11-14). The target hook is rotated and embedded into the articular cartilage at this point and held in place with slight traction while the guide barrel arm of the jig is attached. The thumb should be hyperextended to displace the trapezium dorsally on the

distal articular surface of the scaphoid. The jig is compressed against the scaphoid, seating the guide barrel on the distal articular surface of the scaphoid (Fig. 11-15*A*).

The scale on the jig indicates the appropriate length for the primary guide wire. After the wire has been drilled through the guide barrel and across the fracture, its satisfactory position should be confirmed radiographically (Fig. 11-15*B*). A secondary wire is then measured to length and drilled through the jig across the fracture to control rotation of the fracture fragments during preparation for the screw (Fig. 11-15*C,D*).

The articular cartilage and subchondral bone of the distal pole are broached with a cannulated instrument, and the distal and proximal scaphoid fragments are drilled with an appropriate length cannulated step drill. The cannulated Herbert–Whipple screw is then inserted over the primary guide wire, securing compression of the fracture fragments (Fig. 11-16). The secondary wire may be left in place for 2 weeks if desired to provide additional rotational control. The jig is removed, the scaphotrapezial joint capsule is closed, and the skin edges are approximated.

Postoperative treatment consists of a short-arm

(text continues on page 156)

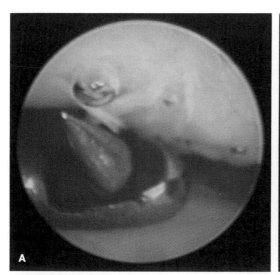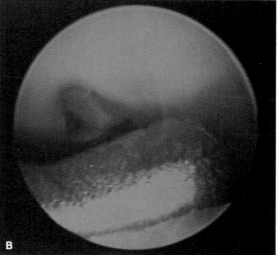

FIGURE 11–14.
(**A**) The intraarticular target hook of jig for a Herbert–Whipple screw. (**B**) The hook is guided arthroscopically to the dorsal proximal aspect of the scaphoid adjacent to the scapholunate ligament, where the hook engages the articular cartilage and bone on the proximal fragment. Viewed through the 3-4 portal (right wrist).

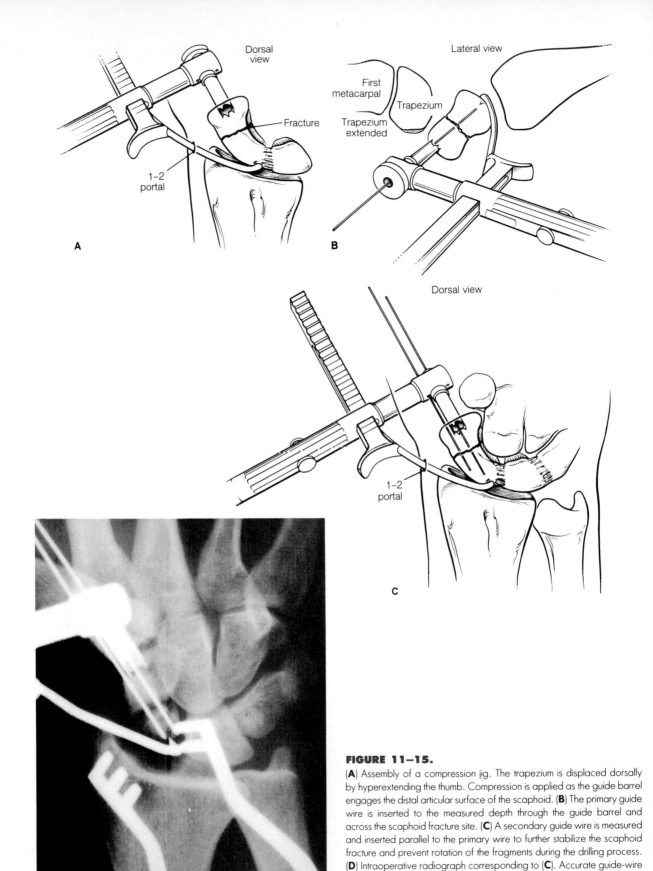

Dorsal
view

Fracture

1–2
portal

A

Lateral view

First
metacarpal   Trapezium

Trapezium
extended

B

Dorsal view

1–2
portal

C

D

FIGURE 11–15.

(**A**) Assembly of a compression jig. The trapezium is displaced dorsally by hyperextending the thumb. Compression is applied as the guide barrel engages the distal articular surface of the scaphoid. (**B**) The primary guide wire is inserted to the measured depth through the guide barrel and across the scaphoid fracture site. (**C**) A secondary guide wire is measured and inserted parallel to the primary wire to further stabilize the scaphoid fracture and prevent rotation of the fragments during the drilling process. (**D**) Intraoperative radiograph corresponding to (**C**). Accurate guide-wire placement should be assured at this stage radiographically. The jig and wires can be repositioned if necessary.

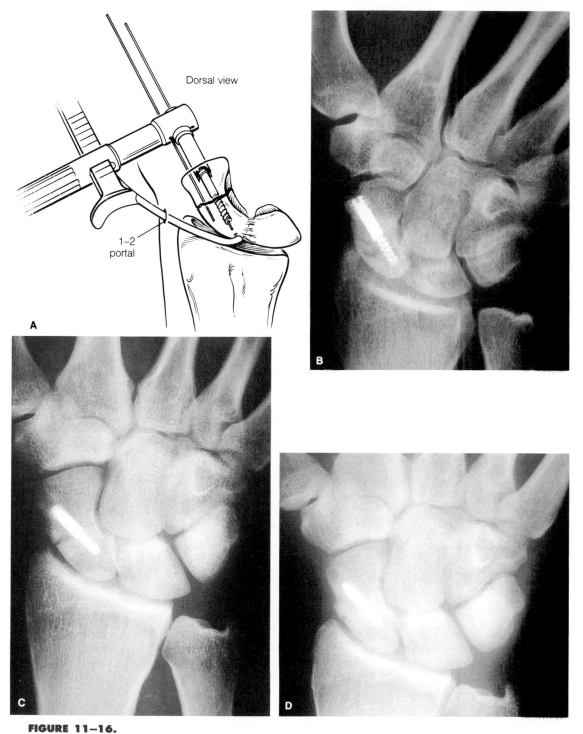

FIGURE 11–16.
(**A**) After drilling over the primary guide wire, an appropriate length Herbert–Whipple cannulated screw is introduced through the guide barrel, transfixing the scaphoid fracture. Compression is maintained by the jig, and rotation is prevented by the secondary wire. (**B**) Screw placement 2 weeks postoperatively. (**C**) Healing progress 6 weeks postoperatively. (**D**) United fracture 10 weeks postoperatively.

cast or volar plaster splint for 4 weeks. Thereafter motion is permitted, but stress, power grip, and loading of the wrist should be avoided until radiographic evidence of fracture union. Alternatively, a functional limited-range splint (DonJoy, Carlsbad, CA) can be applied to block flexion but permit extension.

Early experience with this technique has demonstrated rapid fracture healing and the benefits of much earlier mobilization and return to function than would otherwise be possible.

REFERENCES

1. Herbert TJ. The fractured scaphoid. St. Louis: Quality Medical, 1990.

BIBLIOGRAPHY

Axelrod TS, Paley D, Green J, McMurtry RY. Limited open reduction of the lunate facet and comminuted intraarticular fractures of the distal radius. J Hand Surg [Am] 1988;13(3):372.

Axelrod TS, McMurtry RY. Open reduction and internal fixation of comminuted, intraarticular fractures of the distal radius. J Hand Surg [Am] 1990;15(1):1.

Bartosh RA, Saldana MJ. Intraarticular fractures of the distal radius: a cadaveric study to determine if ligamentotaxis restores radial palmar tilt. J Hand Surg [Am] 1990;15(1):18.

Bennett GL, Leeson MC, Smith BS. Intramedullary fixation of unstable distal radius fractures: a method of fixation allowing early motion. Orthop Rev 1989; 18(2):210.

Bradway JK, Amadio PC, Cooney WP III. Open reduction and internal fixation of displaced comminuted intraarticular fractures of the distal end of the radius. J Bone Joint Surg [Am] 1989;71(6):839.

Burgess RC. The effect of a simulated scaphoid malunion on wrist motion J Hand Surg [Am] 1987;12(5):774.

Cooney WP III, Bussey R, Dobyns JH, Linscheid RL. Difficult wrist fractures: perilunate fracture-dislocations of the wrist. Clin Orthop 1987;(214):136.

Cooney WB III, Dobyns JH, Linscheid RL. Fractures of the scaphoid: a rationale approach to management. Clin Orthop 1980;(149):90.

Cooney WB III, Dobyns JH, Linscheid RL. Non-union of the scaphoid: analysis of the results from bone grafting. J Hand Surg [Am] 1980;5(4):343.

Dobyns JH, Linscheid RL, Cooney WB III. Fractures and locations of the wrist and hand: then and now. J Hand Surg [Am] 1983;8(5):687.

Foster DE, Kopta JA. Update on external fixators in the treatment of wrist fractures. Clin Orthop 1986;(204): 177.

Herbert TJ, Fisher WE. Management of the fractured scaphoid using a new bone screw. J Bone Joint Surg [Br] 1984;66(1):114.

Ipsen T, Larsen CF. A case of scaphocapitate fracture. Acta Orthop Scand 1985;56(6):509.

Jaroma H, Suomalainen O, Hannikainen E, Maki-Kokkila H. Surgical treatment for nonunion of the carpal scaphoid. Ann Chir Gynacecol 1985;(5):239.

Leung KS, Shen WY, Tsang HK, Chiu KH, Leung PC, Hung LK. An effective treatment of comminuted fractures of the distal radius. J Hand Surg [Am] 1990; 15(1):11.

Leyshon A, Ireland J, Trickey EL. The treatment of delayed union and nonunion of the carpal scaphoid by screw fixation. J Bone Joint Surg [Br] 1984;66(1):124.

Light TR. Salvage of intraarticular malunions of the hand and wrist: the role of realignment osteotomy. Clin Orthop 1987;(214):130.

Nakata RY, Chand Y, Matiko JD, Frykman GK, Wood VE. External fixators for wrist fractures: a biomechanical and clinical study. J Hand Surg [Am] 1985; 10(6):845.

Smith DK, Cooney WP III, An KN, Linscheid RL, Chao EY. The effects of simulated unstable scaphoid fractures on carpal motion. J Hand Surg [Am] 1989;14(2): 283.

Smith RS, Crick JC, Alonso J, Horowitz M. Open reduction and internal fixation of volar lip fractures of the distal radius. J Orthop Trauma 1988;2(3):181.

Vance RM, Gelberman RH, Evans EF. Scaphocapitate fractures: patterns of dislocation, mechanisms of injury, and preliminary results of treatment. J Bone Joint Surg [Am] 1980;62(2):271.

Watson HK, Castle TH Jr. Trapezoidal osteotomy of the distal radius for unacceptable articular angulation after Colle's fracture. J Hand Surg [Am] 1988;13(6):837.

Watson HK. Degenerative change in symptomatic scaphoid non-union. J Hand Surg [Am] 1987;12(4): 514.

Zemel NP. The prevention and treatment of complications from fractures of the distal radius and ulna. Hand Clin 1987;3(1):1.

12

Endoscopic Carpal Tunnel Release

James C. Y. Chow

Carpal tunnel syndrome has been studied since 1854, when Sir James Paget described median nerve compression in a patient's wrist following a fracture of the distal radius.[1] In 1880 James Putnam, a Boston neurologist, described symptoms suffered by a group of his patients that today would be diagnosed as carpal tunnel syndrome. In 1913 Marie and Foix, at the autopsy of a patient with advanced atrophy of the thenar muscle and no history of injury, demonstrated neuromata in both median nerves just proximal to the transverse carpal ligament. This was the first recommended decompression of the median nerve by sectioning the transverse carpal ligament to prevent paralysis of the thenar muscles.

Surgical release of the transcarpal ligament for posttraumatic median nerve compression was performed in 1933 by Sir James Learmonth. Cannon and Love reported on 38 cases of tardy median nerve palsy in 1946. This was the first carpal tunnel release for spontaneous median nerve compression in the carpal tunnel. In 1947 Lord Brain and his colleague Wilkinson, together with surgeon Dixon Wright, published the first paper describing in detail the clinical signs, diagnosis, and pathophysiology of spontaneous median nerve compression in the carpal tunnel.[1] Based on their findings, Brain, Wilkinson, and Wright recommended early operative release of the transverse carpal ligament.[1] Before that, the cause of this very common patient complaint was often a mystery for the physician.

As late as 1950, only 12 surgical releases of transcarpal ligament for patients with idiopathic carpal tunnel syndrome were reported.[1] The delay of this compression neuropathy can be attributed both to the confusion caused by diverse manifestations of the median nerve compression in the carpal tunnel and to early investigations of the shoulder and elbow. It was in the 1950s that George Phalen made median nerve decompression of the wrist a well-known procedure with a series of articles on carpal tunnel syndrome, describing what is known today as Tinel's and Phalen's signs.[2-4]

ANATOMY OF THE CARPAL LIGAMENT

The transverse carpal ligament is formed by the deep fascia of the forearm, which is made up of compacted collagen fibers. It has transverse thickening and is attached at both ends to the local bone prominence. The ligament retains the tendons passing under it and is part of the osteofibrous channel. The transverse carpal ligament extends across the hollow on the palmar side of the wrist joint and is attached to the prominence of the trapezium and the scaphoid on the radial side. On the ulnar side, it is attached to the pisiform, the hook of hamate, and the pisohamate ligament. This forms a roof over the transverse arch of the carpal bones, creating a canal called the carpal tunnel. During dissection it is possible to find two distinct layers: a superficial layer attached to the tubercle of the scaphoid and trapezium bones, and a deep layer attached to the medial lip of the groove on the trapezium. Guyon's canal is formed on the ulnar side of the hook of hamate, between the two layers of the fibers. It contains the ulnar nerve, ulnar artery, and vein. The carpal tunnel extends 4 cm beyond the distal crease of the wrist. The osteofibrous carpal tunnel is a constricted zone designed to contain nine flexor tendons in the synovial sheath and to permit their movement during flexion of the wrist. The principal sources of blood supply to the transverse carpal ligament can be divided into superficial and deep. The superficial network is formed by branches of the ulnar artery; the deep network of branches is formed by the palmar superficial arch.

PATHOGENESIS OF CARPAL TUNNEL SYNDROME

The term carpal tunnel syndrome now applies to all conditions producing irritation and/or compression of the median nerve within the carpal canal. The median nerve may be directly damaged or secondarily compressed by any condition that decreases the space. Conditions that reduce the capacity of the carpal tunnel and produce symptoms include the following: deformed Colle's fracture, edema from the tendon sheath, any soft-tissue tumor in the canal, and increased thickness of the carpal ligament itself. Many other systemic conditions such as obesity, diabetes, thyroid dysfunctions, Raynaud's disease, scleroderma, the last trimester of pregnancy, rheumatoid disease, kidney disease under dialysis, acute lupus erythematosus, or other collagen disease also can be related to this syndrome.

DIAGNOSIS

Since carpal tunnel syndrome is a subjective condition, the patient's history is very important. Patients usually complain of paresthesia, which is described as tingling and numbness over the median nerve distribution of the hand. Characteristically it is nocturnal. These symptoms can develop into a referred pain to the forearm and upper arm. The patient usually relieves the symptoms by allowing the hand to drop to the side of the bed, by shaking the hand, or by wriggling the fingers. As the condition progresses, the patient may wake up several times during a single night and get very little sleep as a result.

Carpal tunnel syndrome can be divided into three stages: early, progressive, and late. In the early stages, the symptoms appear only when provoked and are related to specific activities. The symptoms are mainly sensory without motor involvement. In the progressive stage, sensory findings are more advanced, and motor weakness begins to occur in the affected hand. The patient begins to wake up at night, the classic symptom of carpal tunnel syndrome. Patients usually seek medical assistance when symptoms suddenly become worse and disturb their daily functioning. In the late stage, patients have usually had these symptoms for many years, with moderate muscle weakness including thenar muscle atrophy. Patients in the advanced stage may report that at one point in the past the intolerable symptoms became somewhat better. The condition, however, is not actually improving, but permanent median nerve damage has resulted in less complaints from the patient. These patients sometimes have no response in the sensory or motor distal latency on the nerve conductive test. Patients may become asymptomatic to pain and tingling, but a persistent numbness indicates permanent nerve damage.

On physical examination, the patient experiences paresthesia or a decrease in sensation. Symptoms are always most pronounced on the median nerve distribution, whereas the small fingers are never involved in a typical median nerve compression syndrome. Light percussion over the median nerve at the wrist produces Tinel's sign, a tingling sensation radiating to the long fingers. Phalen's sign, or the wrist flexion test, is observed by having the patient hold the forearm vertically and dropping both hands into complete flexion at the wrist. In this position, the median nerve is squeezed between the proximal edge of the transcarpal ligament, the adjacent flexor tendons, and the radius. If a numbness and tingling is produced over the median nerve distribution of the hand within 60 seconds, the finding is positive.

In the late stages of the syndrome, thenar muscle atrophy and weakness of pinch and grip occurs in the involved hand. This is usually associated with dropping things, spilling coffee, and an inability to pick up fine objects from smooth surfaces. Electromyography (EMG) and nerve conduction velocity (NCV) tests help illustrate the delay of the distal latencies of the nerve in the transcarpal canal. A careful examination should be done by the physician to exclude the possibility of a cervical disc, the thoracic outlet syndrome, and other central nervous system conditions. Wrist radiographs should include AP, lateral, and carpal tunnel views. This is necessary to exclude any bone or joint deformities, abnormalities, or pathologies. If more extensive study is indicated, it should include magnetic resonance imaging, computed tomography scans, bone scans, and an arthrogram of the wrist.

CONSERVATIVE TREATMENT

Surgical treatment is not required for every patient with carpal tunnel syndrome, and conservative treatment usually is required first. Nonsteroidal antiinflammatory oral medication, night-splinting of the affected hand, resting the hand, antivibration work gloves, and a change in occupation are advised in the early and progressive stage patient. Steroid injection in the carpal canal sometimes gives relief from symptoms; 1 ml or less of hydrocortisone (Celestrone, 6 mg) can be injected using a 25-gauge

needle just medial to the palmaris longus tendon. This steroid can be combined with a local anesthetic. Care must be taken not to inject the steroid solution into the median nerve itself, but rather to disperse the solution around the flexor tendons. Additional injections should not be given more frequently than 7 to 10 days apart. If symptoms recur after 3 or 4 injections, surgical intervention is advised. If thenar muscle atrophy is present or the patient's symptoms are of long duration, injection is seldom of value, and surgical treatment should be recommended immediately.

SURGICAL TREATMENT

The standard open surgical procedure is a longitudinal curved incision in the palm, ulnar to and parallel to the thenar crease. If necessary, the cut can be extended proximal to the flexor crease of the wrist, forming a lazy S-shaped incision. (This extended cut should form a curve or an angle to the flexor crease because a straight cut across the crease can form a painful scar postoperatively.) The deep structures are exposed and the carpal ligament is released under direct vision. Following surgery, a compression dressing, volar splint, or both are usually applied.

Another surgical technique uses a transverse incision over the distal wrist crease. The incision is approximately 5 cm in length and involves a blind cut toward the carpal ligament. The danger of this technique is in either cutting too far distally, which increases the chance of injuring the digital nerve and the superficial palmar artery, or undercutting and not completely releasing the carpal ligament. Most surgeons have recommended abandoning this method.

ENDOSCOPIC RELEASE OF THE CARPAL LIGAMENT

Only recently has arthroscopic technique been applied to the wrist area in an attempt to release the carpal ligament. These attempts have been made because of successful results with knee arthroscopy, including decreased postoperative pain, diminished scarring, and a quicker recovery with less discomfort to the patient. Three techniques will be described in this chapter: the method of Okutsu and colleagues, or the Japanese technique;[5,6] Agee's technique;* and Chow's technique.[7,8]

Japanese Technique

The Japanese technique involves a transverse incision over the volar surface of the wrist. A dull, blunt plastic tube is passed along the ulnar side of the palmaris longus, and the arthroscope is introduced inside the tube. The structures visible through the tube include the carpal ligament. An unprotected hook knife passes along the ulnar side of the plastic tube. The distal end of the carpal ligament is identified and hooked with the hook knife. It is then retracted proximally to release the carpal ligament. This requires several passes to release the ligament completely. In their early report, one recurrence and several hematomas of the wrist were recorded with no other complications. I have had no experience with this technique.

Agee's Technique

Dr. Agee from California describes a different endoscopic release of the carpal ligament. His technique requires an incision that closely resembles the standard transverse incision over the wrist. However, instead of cutting blindly, he designed a special pistol-shaped instrument (Fig. 12-1). The arthroscope and camera are hooked to the back of the pistol, and the tip of the pistol has an open window through which one can view. A blade controlled by the trigger is designed on the distal end.

As with any procedure with limited exposure, precautions are necessary to avoid injury to crucial nerves and vessels.

After tourniquet and routine skin preparation, make a transverse incision in the proximal wrist flexion crease from the palmaris longus to the flexor carpi ulnaris. Expose the volar carpal ligament, and

_____
Agee FM, personal communication, September, 1990.

cut a distal flap in the ligament in line with the ring finger. Lift the flap, and scrape the fat and synovium from the dorsal surface of the transverse carpal ligament with a narrow elevator. Dilate the entrance to the canal with specially designed probes.

Next, insert the scope and sheath deep into the transverse carpal ligament, aiming toward the ring finger and viewing upward at the dorsal surface of the ligament. A fatty mass marks the distal end of the ligament and envelopes the proximal palmar arterial arch. Deploy the blade proximal to this fatty mass. Maintain lifting pressure on the scope sheath and withdraw the instrument, dividing the transverse carpal ligament. More than one pass may be necessary for a chronically thick ligament. When completely incised, the edges of the transverse carpal ligament will spring apart.

Divide the volar carpal ligament subcutaneously with scissors proximal to the incision. Apply skin closure and a soft dressing with or without splinting. The incision usually is sealed within 5 days because the skin is flexible, mobile, and well-vascularized at the wrist. Activity is then permitted according to comfort.

Experience with this procedure is limited, but indications are that it effectively decompresses the median nerve, eliminates the palmar incision, and can safely avoid injury to the nerve, its motor branch, the palmar cutaneous branch, and the proximal palmar arch. Modifications to the instrumentation may be necessary to further reduce risk of injury to the digital nerves.

Chow's Technique

The major differences between Chow's technique and the two endoscopic techniques described above are as follows:

Two arthroscopic portals are used rather than one incision. Each portal measures approximately ½ inch or 1 cm in length.
A single pass is required to establish the position, which is secured with a slotted tube. The arthroscope is brought in after this position is achieved.
The knife that resects the ligament is completely protected by the tube until cutting begins.

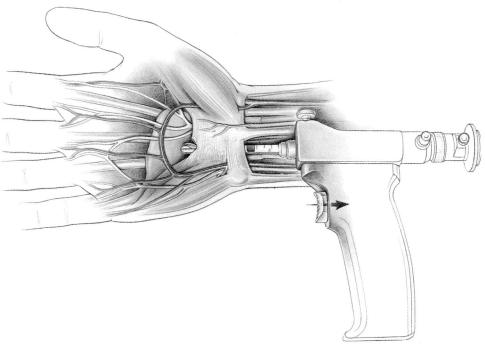

FIGURE 12–1.

Agee's technique for endoscopic carpal tunnel release. The blade is deployed distal to the transverse carpal ligament and proximal to the transverse palmar arch. Ligament is cut as instrument is withdrawn in a proximal direction.

Numerous cuts can be made until the resection meets the surgeon's satisfaction.

The cutting is all under direct vision. The only complication reported with this technique was a temporary ulnar nerve palsy in two patients, one of whom recovered spontaneously in 4 weeks and one who recovered more slowly.

Setup

The patient is placed in the supine position, and the hand table is used for the involved hand. Two video monitors are used, one facing the surgeon and one facing the assistant. A monitor may also be viewed by the patient as it is usually located on the opposite side of surgical hand. The surgeon sits on the axillary or ulnar side of the patient, and the assistant faces the surgeon.

Anesthesia

Local anesthesia plus intravenous medication is recommended so that the surgeon can communicate with the patient. An alert patient can inform the surgeon of a variation in the nerve structure. One percent Xylocaine Without Epinephrine is used at the entry and exit portals. One to two milligrams of 1 mg/ml intravenous Versed is given prior to making the surgical incision. Before the insertion of the slotted/conical abdurator assembly, 100–150 μg of 500 μg/ml Alfenta (alfentanil hydrochloride) is given intravenously. This analgesia is usually adequate and allows the patient to tolerate the procedure quite well. Immediately after the procedure, the surgeon can examine the patient while still in a sterilized environment. If any complications have occurred which may necessitate a second procedure (*e.g.,* tendon repair, nerve repair), it can be performed immediately.

Entry Portal

The proximal end of the pisiform bone is palpated with the fingertip. A circle approximately ¼ cm in diameter is drawn. This covers only the proximal end of the pisiform. Starting from the center of the small circle, a line is drawn approximately 1 cm radially; from the end of that line a second line is drawn 1 cm proximally. Starting at the end of the second line, a third line is drawn radially about 1 cm. This line is the entry portal, and it is usually located on the ulnar side of the palmaris longus and the radial side of the ulnar neurovascular bundle. The incision is just on top of the flexor tendon. The ulnar artery is palpable with the fingers, and the incision should be radial from that position.

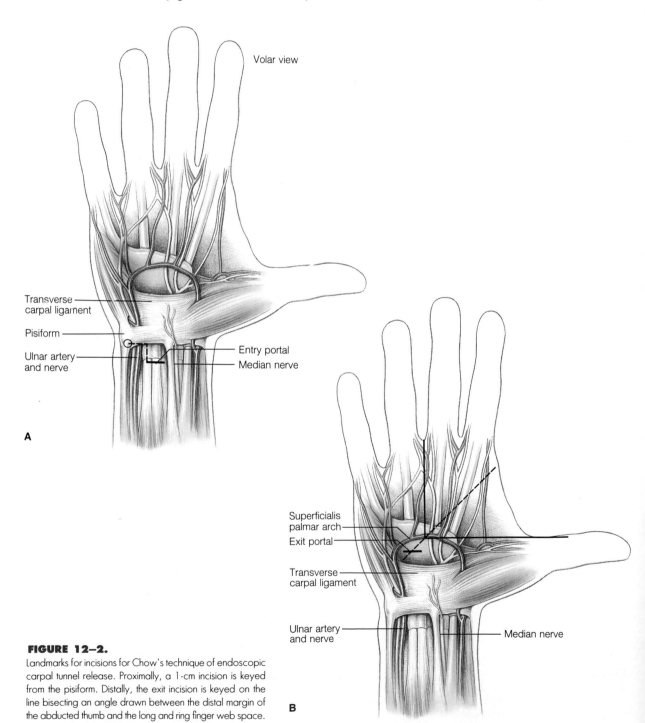

FIGURE 12–2.
Landmarks for incisions for Chow's technique of endoscopic carpal tunnel release. Proximally, a 1-cm incision is keyed from the pisiform. Distally, the exit incision is keyed on the line bisecting an angle drawn between the distal margin of the abducted thumb and the long and ring finger web space.

Exit Portal

With the thumb in full abduction, a line is drawn from the distal border of the thumb. This line will meet with the line drawn at the third web space, which is the space between the middle and ring fingers. Those two lines usually form a right angle. The exit portal should be located on the bisect line of this right angle, which is approximately 1 cm from the junction of those two lines. After the tip of the trocar is palpated subcutaneously, the exit portal is made. A variable of 1 mm from the point drawn is acceptable (Fig. 12-2).

Insertion of the Chow's Slotted Tube

One percent lidocaine (Xylocaine) is injected into both the entry and exit portals. A 1-cm transverse incision is made for the entry portal. A hemostat is used for blunt dissection, and the superficial vein is pushed away to avoid bleeding. The fascia is opened longitudinally. If bleeding occurs at this time, a tourniquet should be applied, since a clear view is crucial to this dissection. After the fascia is cut, the ulnar bursa will be seen. Two dissectors are used; the curved dissector is usually held toward the finger, and the straight dissector is held proximally. It is very important to open the bursa completely. Otherwise, the ulnar neurovascular bundle will most likely be retracted toward the flexor tendon, increasing the chance of damage to the ulnar neurovascular bundle, especially the ulnar nerve. After the bursa is opened, the flexor tendons and the tendon sheath can be seen. The flexor tendons can be retracted radially, one at a time, without entry to the tendon sheath until the entire group is retracted radially. At this time, a space between the flexor tendons and the ulnar neurovascular bundle should be identified (Fig. 12-3). The straight dissector can easily be passed into the carpal canal. The patient

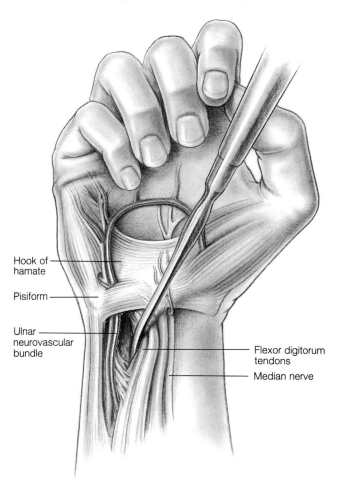

Hook of hamate

Pisiform

Ulnar neurovascular bundle

Flexor digitorum tendons

Median nerve

FIGURE 12–3.
Identification of the space between the ulnar neurovascular bundle and the flexor digitorum superficialis tendons is made before inserting the endoscope trocar and sheath.

sometimes complains of discomfort when the blunt trocar touches the floor of the wrist area. To relieve discomfort, 100–150 μg intravenous Alfenta can be given by the anesthesiologist. If the trocar meets any resistance, the location may be incorrect. The procedure should be stopped immediately and dissection begun again. The space between the flexor tendon and the ulnar neurovascular bundle is easily identified, and the trocar can be inserted without any resistance. Great caution must be exercised to protect the neurovascular bundle. At times pulsation of the ulnar artery can be seen. The tip of the trocar will touch the base of the hook of hamate, and, following the body of the hook of hamate, is lifted upward (Fig. 12-4). The tip of the assembly will touch the carpal ligament. With the finger and wrist

in full extension, the trocar is advanced distally. As soon as the trocar passes through the carpal ligament, the tip should enter the subcutaneous tissue, usually coming within a millimeter of the exit portal that was previously marked. A small transverse incision is made, and the trocar is advanced through the exit portal. The hand is stabilized with a special holder and strap (Fig. 12-5). The arthroscope is then introduced.

ENDOSCOPIC EXAMINATION

The tension created by hyperextending the hand and the round geometry of the sheath assembly causes the flexor tendons and other tissues to fall

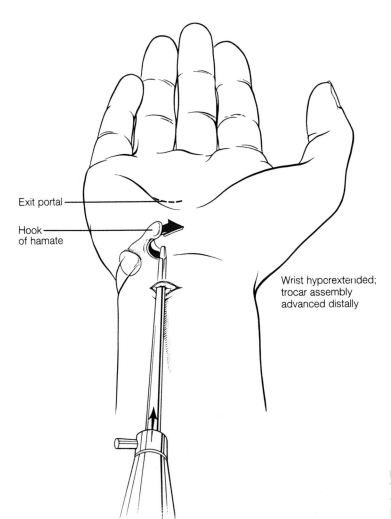

Exit portal

Hook of hamate

Wrist hyperextended; trocar assembly advanced distally

FIGURE 12–4.
With the wrist hyperextended, the endoscopy sheath and trocar are advanced to touch the base of the hook of hamate.

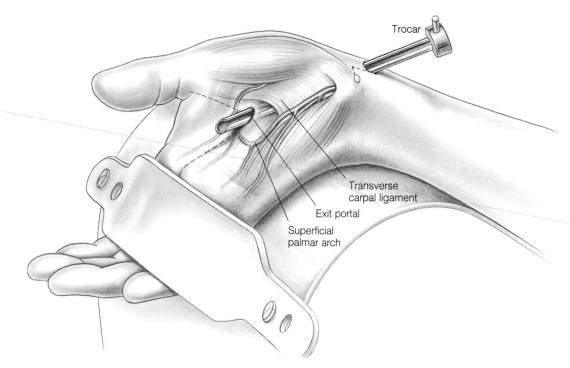

Trocar

Transverse
carpal ligament

Exit portal

Superficial
palmar arch

FIGURE 12—5.
A stabilizing frame for hyperextension of the wrist and fingers to retract flexor tendons dorsally within the carpal canal.

away from the sheath assembly as it advances distally. Further hyperextension of the wrist and fingers ensures that the obturator remains superior to the superficial palmar arch (Fig. 12-6).

Insert the arthroscope proximally into the sheath. With a blunt hook probe, dissect the thin bursal membrane that is sometimes seen covering the sheath's slotted opening. If fogging or material obscures vision, a swab can be used to clear the field of view. The swab is inserted and rotated radially.

Identify the carpal ligament. Carpal ligament fibers usually run transversely and can be clearly seen (Fig. 12-7). A white swollen piece of tissue running longitudinally on the radial side of the opening is

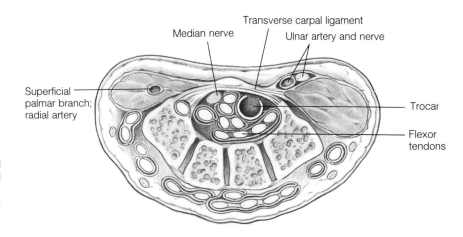

Median nerve

Transverse carpal ligament

Ulnar artery and nerve

Superficial
palmar branch;
radial artery

Trocar

Flexor
tendons

FIGURE 12—6.
A transverse section through the carpal canal shows the location of the slotted endoscope sheath superficial to the tendons found immediately beneath the transverse carpal ligaments.

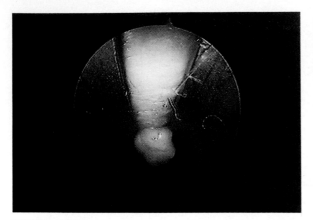

FIGURE 12–7.
Transverse fibers of the deep surface of the transverse carpal ligament.

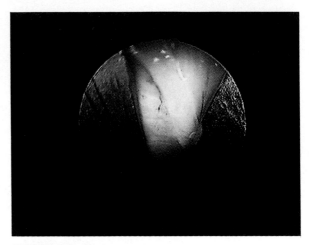

FIGURE 12–8.
An overhanging edge of the flexor tendon bursa on the radial side of the slotted endoscope sheath.

either the ulnar edge of the median nerve or the flexor tendon bursa (Fig. 12-8). Rotate the sheath 5° to 10° toward the ulnar side to protect this structure from inadvertent injury. Probe the sheath distally to proximally until the entire width of the carpal ligament is clearly seen. No other tissue should be visible between the sheath and the carpal ligament. If in doubt, reinsert the conical obturator, remove the sheath assembly, and begin again.

LIGAMENT CUTTING TECHNIQUE

First, release the distal edge of the carpal ligament (Fig. 12-9*A*). With the arthroscope proximal in the sheath, insert the forward probe knife into the distal opening. The design of this knife permits forward cutting only. The knife's blunt proximal surface can be used to safely probe proximally to distally along the ligament. The cutting edge is used to release the distal edge of the ligament, cutting distally to proximally. Cutting in this direction keeps the knife within the safety zone.

Next, cut through the midsection of the carpal ligament with a triangle knife (Fig. 12-9*B*). The design of the triangular blade allows a controlled upward cut.

Gently insert the blunt tip of the retrograde knife through the opening just made with the triangular knife. Draw the sharp proximal cutting edge of the retrograde knife distally, joining the first two cuts, and completely releasing the distal aspect of the carpal ligament (Fig. 12-9*C*).

Remove the endoscope from the proximal opening of the sheath and place it into the distal opening. Probe the sheath, identifying the previous cut and proximal edge of the carpal ligament. Use the forward probe knife to cut the proximal edge of the ligament (Fig. 12-9*D*). The retrograde knife is then used to completely release the proximal aspect of the ligament (Fig. 12-9*E*). Meticulously examine the area endoscopically both proximally and distally to ensure that the carpal ligament has been fully released. Should further resection be required, choose the appropriate knife to complete the release.

Insert the conical obturator into the sheath, and remove the sheath. Usually a single suture suffices to close the incisions. Apply pressure for 2 to 3 minutes to stop any bleeding (usually there is none), and apply a simple dressing that leaves the fingers and thumb free to move.

Postoperative Treatment

Active exercise begins immediately after surgery. The patient is advised to avoid heavy lifting or pushing down on the palm until the discomfort disappears, usually for 2 to 3 weeks. If the patient engages in heavy lifting activities too soon, it may result in some swelling and prolonged pain in the palm area. The sutures are removed in 1 week to 10 days.

Based on clinical results, I believe that the carpal

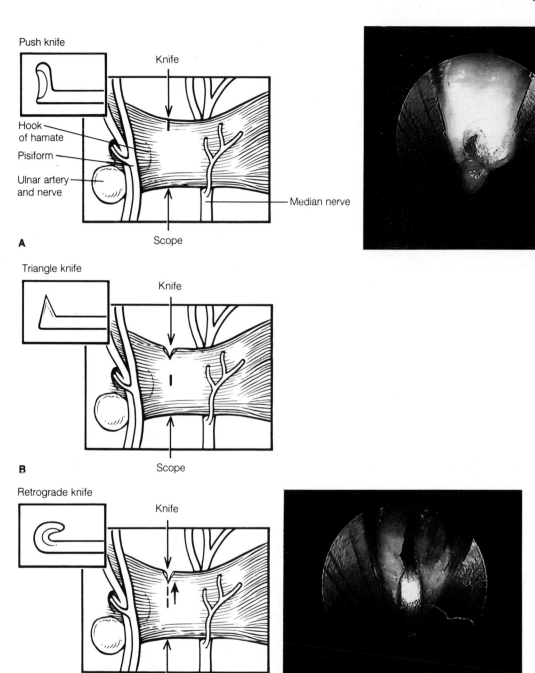

FIGURE 12—9.

A sequence of cuts is used to divide the transverse carpal ligament. (**A**) The push knife cuts the distal edge of the ligament. (**B**) The triangle knife punctures the midportion of the ligament. (**C**) The retrograde knife connects cut **B** with cut **A**. (**D**) The push knife initiates cut on the proximal edge of the ligament. (**E**) The retrograde knife connects cuts **B** and **D**, completing the transection of the transverse carpal ligament.

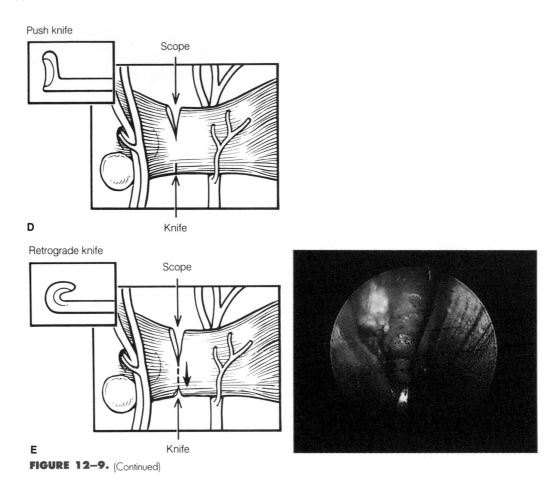

FIGURE 12—9. (Continued)

ligament does not have a rich blood or nerve fiber supply, so that cutting the ligament alone and bypassing the other tissues definitely decreases postoperative pain, bleeding, and scarring. The palmaris longus tendon expansion and the muscle fibers are also preserved by endoscopic technique, which prevents the bowstringing of the flexor tendon. By preserving the continuation of the thenar and lesser thenar muscle fibers, it also preserves the pinch and grip strength. Whether this technique increases the chance of recurrence is yet to be seen.

The best results with carpal tunnel syndrome decompression have been obtained in patients who have had symptoms for a short time. This may be because the initial recoverable neuropathy is succeeded by more permanent changes in the nerve. The less invasive endoscopic carpal tunnel release may change the future treatment of carpal tunnel syndrome because the patient will not be facing a long recovery and disability as is common with the standard open procedure.

I would like to thank my wife, Ada, for her assistance in the preparation of this chapter.

REFERENCES

1. Pfeffer GB, Gelberman RH, Boyes JH, Rydevik B. The history of carpal tunnel syndrome. J Hand Surg [Br] 1988;13:28
2. Phalen GS, Gardner W, Lalonde A. Neuropathy of the median nerve due to compression beneath the transverse carpal ligament. J Bone Joint Surg [Am] 1950;32:109.
3. Phalen GS. The carpal tunnel syndrome: seventeen years experience in diagnosis and treatment of six hundred fifty-four hands. J Bone Joint Surg [Am] 1966;48:211.

4. Phalen GS, Kendrick J, Rodriguez J. Lipomas of the upper extremity. Am J Surg 1971;121:298.

5. Okutsu I, Ninomiya S, Takatori Y, Ugawa Y. Endoscopic management of carpal tunnel syndrome. Arthroscopy 1989;5:11.

6. Okutsu I, Ninomiya S, Hamanaka I, Kuroshima N, Inanami H. Measurement of pressure in the carpal canal before and after endoscopic management of carpal tunnel syndrome. J Bone Joint Surg [Am] 1989;71: 679.

7. Chow CY. Endoscopic release of the carpal ligament: a new technique for carpal tunnel syndrome. Arthroscopy 1989;5:19.

8. Chow CY. Endoscopic release of the carpal ligament for carpal tunnel syndrome: 22 month clinical result. Arthroscopy 1990;6:288.

BIBLIOGRAPHY

Barr WG, Blair SJ. Carpal tunnel syndrome as the initial manifestation of scleroderma. J Hand Surg [Am] 1988;13:366.

Bloem JJ, Pradiarahardja CL, Vuursteen PJ. The post-carpal tunnel syndrome: causes and prevention. Neth J Surg 1986;38(2):52.

Eiken O, Carstam N, Eddeland A. Anomalous distal branching of the median nerve. Scand J Plast Reconstr Surg Hand Surg 1971;5:149.

Entin MA. Carpal tunnel syndrome and its variants. Surg Clin North Am 1968;48:1097.

Gelberman RH, Hergenroeder PT, Hargens AR, Lundborg GN, Akeson WH. The carpal tunnel syndrome: a study of carpal canal pressures. J Bone Joint Surg [Am] 1981;63:380.

Gelberman RH, Pfeffer GB, Galbraith RT, Szabo RM, Rydevik B, Dimick M. Results of treatment of severe carpal-tunnel syndrome without internal neurolysis of the median nerve. J Bone Joint Surg [Am] 1987;69: 896.

Kerrigan JJ, Bertoni JM, Jaeger SH. Ganglion cysts and carpal tunnel syndrome. J Hand Surg [Am] 1988;13: 763.

Kleinert J. The nerve of Henle. J Hand Surg [Am] 1990;15:784.

Kremchek TE, Kremchek EJ. Carpal tunnel syndrome caused by flexor tendon sheath lipoma. Orthop Rev 1988;17:1083.

Langloh ND, Linscheid RL. Recurrent and unrelieved carpal-tunnel syndrome. Clin Orthop Relat Res 1972;83:41.

Lanz U. Anatomical variations of the median nerve in the carpal tunnel. J Hand Surg [Am] 1977;2:44.

Louis DS, Greene TL, Noellert RC. Complications of carpal tunnel surgery. J Neurosurg 1985;62:3526.

Lowry WE, Follender AB. Interfascicular neurolysis in the severe carpal tunnel syndrome. Clin Orthop 1988;227:251.

Mannerfelt L, Hybbinette CH. Important anomaly of the thenar motor branch of the median nerve. Bull Hosp Jt Dis Orthop Inst 1972;33:15.

Papathanassiou BT. A variant of the motor branch of the median nerve in the hand. J Bone Joint Surg [Br] 1968;50:156.

Rhoades CE, Gelberman RH, Szabo RM, Botte M. The results of carpal tunnel release with and without internal neurolysis of the median nerve for severe carpal tunnel release. J Hand Surg [Am] 1986;11:448.

Richman JG, Gelberman R, Rydevik B, Gylys-Morin V. Carpal tunnel volume determination by magnetic imaging three-dimensional reconstruction. J Hand Surg [Am] 1987;12:712.

Skie M, Zeiss J, Ebraheim NA, Jackson WT. Carpal tunnel changes and median nerve compression during wrist flexion and extension seen by magnetic resonance imaging. J Hand Surg [Am] 1990;15:934.

13

Precautions and Complications

*F*ortunately, complications associated with arthroscopic surgical procedures are infrequent. Most complications can be avoided with careful attention to surgical detail and prudent general surgical principles. Wrist arthroscopy can be a tedious procedure. It should never be undertaken casually, but rather with diligence, forethought, and adequate preoperative planning. Considerable laboratory practice using joint models or cadaveric specimens is recommended to develop the familiarity and perspective required to recognize and interpret visual fields and to cultivate the gentle fine motor skills necessary for these procedures. A few clinicians will be fortunate enough to have access to supervised clinical training in wrist arthroscopy. With sufficient preoperative preparation and surgical precision, complications can be minimized and patients will be most likely to achieve optimal surgical results.

For discussion purposes, complications can be considered in three categories:

1. Those related to specific tissues
2. Those related to execution of the procedure
3. Those related to recuperation and ultimate therapeutic results.

SPECIFIC TISSUE COMPLICATIONS

Any of the intraarticular or juxtaarticular tissues of the wrist can be injured during the course of an arthroscopic procedure. To avoid this unnecessary surgical trauma, instruments should be introduced and manipulated in a very gentle fashion. The surgeon must always be alert to any resistance or impediment to the movement of instruments within the joint. If resistance is encountered, the surgeon must pause to decipher the cause. Excessive pressure on articular cartilage can easily scuff its fragile surface and cause permanent and irreparable damage to the otherwise smooth and slippery surface. Usually, such injuries are caused by the arthroscope. The contact of its tip or sheath with the articular surface is obscured from the visual field. Without tactile sensitivity, the surgeon may be unaware of excessive pressure on the articular cartilage until the scope is moved and the damage is seen.

Injury to articular cartilage may also occur during introduction of the arthroscope or accessory instruments into the joint. Improperly placed portals will not lead the instruments into the appropriate space. Articular cartilage may be punctured or lacerated by the tip of the instrument (Fig. 13-1). If one is uncertain about the selected portal location, it can be tested by the preliminary introduction of a hypodermic needle. The portal selected should allow the needle to enter unimpeded, parallel with the plane of the articular surface. Sharp trocars are ill-advised, because any inadvertent plunge into the joint or even a gentle twisting motion can lacerate joint surfaces.

If major resistance is encountered on attempts to introduce instruments through the joint capsule, the instrument is probably being directed against bone. In elderly patients or patients who have osteopenia, persistence or even the firm twisting of the instrument or trocar can drill into cortical or subchondral bone. Although these injuries will usually heal, they do cause pain, unnecessary bleeding,

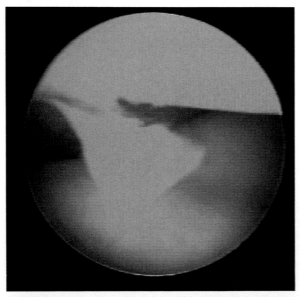

FIGURE 13–1.
Iatrogenic articular cartilage defect from introduction of arthroscope trocar.

and full-thickness injury to the overlying articular cartilage.

Ligaments may be injured if perforated directly in the course of establishing a portal. They can also be partially cut if the scalpel blade is introduced too deeply when lancing the skin. Ligament injuries also will usually heal, but their disruption is completely unnecessary.

The dorsal extensor tendons are usually palpable except for the extensor indicis proprius and the extensor digiti quinti (EDQ). Again, tendon injury in the course of establishing arthroscopy portals is unnecessary if the surgeon pays keen attention to the topographical anatomy, palpating and marking the location of each tendon compartment. Avoiding deep incisions with the scalpel and using only blunt trocars will avert almost any injury to tendons.

Cutaneous nerve branches are also in jeopardy of injury during the establishment of arthroscope portals. The described practice of spreading cutaneous tissue with a fine-point hemostat is an important protective measure. This mobilizes the cutaneous nerve branches and enables them to easily slide or roll out of the way when a blunt instrument is introduced. Again, it is important to avoid deep insertion of the scalpel blade through the skin. Rather, the skin should be pulled against the tip of the scalpel blade when incising the dermis. Neuroma formation is painful and long-lasting, if not permanent.

When C-wires or K-wires are drilled into carpal bones or fracture fragments percutaneously, small defects on the pin surface may capture cutaneous nerve branches in the subcutaneous tissue, severely twisting or avulsing them. This can be avoided by using a pin cannula fashioned from a 14- or 16-gauge needle to protect the subcutaneous tissue when introducing pins.

The most significant vascular structure that must be protected is the radial artery. Knowledge of its very consistent anatomic location and course is imperative. The artery enters the anatomic snuff box by emerging dorsally from beneath the first extensor compartment. It then courses distally in a groove to enter the thumb web space over the dorsal aspect of the first metacarpal base (Fig. 13-2). The 1-2 portal can jeopardize the radial artery if it is not properly placed near the intersection of the extensor carpi radialis longus (ECRL) and the extensor pollicis

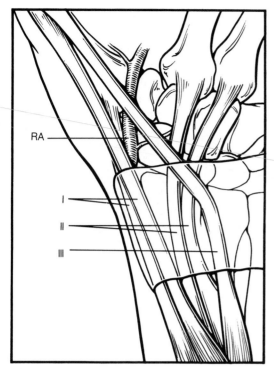

FIGURE 13–2.

Course of the radial artery (RA) in the anatomic snuff box. The artery emerges dorsally from beneath the first extensor compartment and courses distally in a groove to enter the thumb web space over the base of the first metacarpal. I, first extensor compartment; II, second extensor compartment; III, third extensor compartment.

longus (EPL). Maintaining a dorsal position in the snuff box for this portal avoids the radial artery by 6 to 10 mm, depending on the patient's size.

Dorsal veins will usually roll easily in the subcutaneous tissue. Their variable course precludes protecting them completely from inadvertent laceration when incising the skin. However, if the skin is pulled against the scalpel point as recommended, injury to these veins is uncommon and should be inconsequential.

Careful attention should be paid to the condition of the patient's skin. The application and removal of fingertraps can damage certain fragile skin, especially in the presence of predisposing systemic conditions such as rheumatoid arthritis, systemic lupus, or senile atrophy. Flexible nylon fingertraps are more gentle than metal or reed traps. They have very fine edges and a broad surface that distributes compression forces evenly. In the presence of fragile

skin disorders, one should incorporate three or more digits into fingertraps to further distribute the load. The least possible effective traction force should be used, and the length of the procedure should be kept as brief as possible.

Other tissues remotely located from the operative site in the upper extremity are also potentially subject to injury during wrist arthroscopy, further complicating the procedure. Traction injuries to the metacarpophalangeal ligaments are possible, although to my knowledge they have never been encountered or described. It is also conceivable that traction injuries to the brachial plexus or more distal primary nerves could be caused with certain imprudent traction arrangements. Traction applied during anesthesia is always potentially hazardous to nerves, and judicious application and precautions must be used. Attention should also be directed to the ulnar nerve, which is vulnerable to pressure in the cubital tunnel on the back of the elbow. Injury to the ulnar nerve is extremely unlikely because the elbow is usually suspended slightly when traction is applied; however, the ulnar nerve is so sensitive to pressure, the mention of the possibility of injury is necessary.

TECHNICAL COMPLICATIONS OF THE SURGICAL PROCEDURE

In the course of performing any surgical procedure, complications can occur that impede or compromise execution of the procedure. These complications may have transient or lasting effects. The surgeon should know how to correct or neutralize these unexpected contingencies and should always have alternative options in mind.

Bleeding is a notable example. Intraarticular bleeding in the course of any arthroscopic procedure obscures the visual field. Bleeding in the wrist can occur from fracture lines, lacerations of the capsule, or, more rarely, from the margins of an entry portal. It can nearly always be controlled by an experienced assistant who can balance satisfactorily the inflow and outflow rates of irrigating solution. The wrist is a low-volume joint. If bleeding occurs, complete fluid exchange requires only a few milliliters. Suction instruments will frequently overpower inflow mechanisms. The regulators available for wall suction are not sensitive enough to permit precisely regulated flow. The use of a mechanical irrigation pump that monitors intraarticular pressure and flow may be helpful in these situations, but manual pumps or the use of passive outflow will usually suffice.

Imbalance in the inflow and outflow of irrigating solutions may introduce bubbles into the joint. Even the most minute bubbles in this small joint can compromise visibility. The arthroscope cannula and other hollow instruments can always be held inclined distally to allow bubbles to rise toward the extraarticular end of the instrument. If air does enter the joint, it can usually be evacuated easily by inserting a small hypodermic needle through the skin and piercing the bubble (Fig 13-3). The positive intraarticular fluid pressure will evacuate the bubble through the needle.

Finally, one should consider the intraoperative risk of fluid extravasation. Fluid leakage through the capsule around arthroscopic instruments is common. Excessive extravasation into the subcutaneous tissue dorsally can make it impossible to palpate topographical landmarks used to identify needed accessory portal sites. It is principally for this reason that all topographical landmarks should be located and drawn on the skin at the beginning of each procedure. Precise portal location is imperative. Identification of the extensor tendons and the articular margins is the essential guide to portal placement.

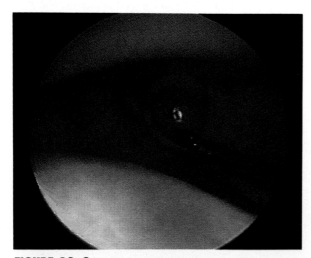

FIGURE 13—3.
An air bubble being evacuated by hypodermic needle.

Extravasation of irrigation fluid into muscle compartments poses minimal risk to the patient. Even in the presence of severely comminuted intraarticular fractures, the extravasation of physiologic irrigating solutions such as Ringer's lactate or normal saline will raise the intracompartmental pressure only briefly. These fluids are absorbed by clisis in a matter of minutes and will not sustain elevated compartmental pressures long enough to compromise circulation and provoke ischemic contracture. Even so, it is advisable to wrap the forearm with a snug compression bandage when operating on acute fractures with elevated intraarticular fluid pressure. This practice will retard extravasation of irritating solution into the muscle compartments.

Perhaps the single most frustrating intraoperative complication is equipment breakage or malfunction. Wrist arthroscopy is an equipment-dependent procedure. There are few instruments that will substitute for those specifically designed for a particular task in this small joint. It is advisable, therefore, to have back-up equipment available—preferably sterile—in the event of any malfunction. Regular instrument inspection, lubrication (if necessary), and testing is invaluable. Otherwise, it may be necessary to terminate an unfinished procedure without significant benefit to the patient, but with unavoidable expense incurred.

Finally, the magnitude of these procedures should not be underestimated to patients. There is always the potential—however small—for anesthetic complications intraoperatively or for physiologic responses that require abortion of the procedure. Fortunately, such occurrences are rare. However, the preparedness for anesthetic complications should never be compromised based on the benignity of the planned surgery.

COMPLICATIONS AFFECTING THERAPEUTIC RESULTS

The ultimate success of most orthopaedic surgical procedures depends to a large extent on perioperative events. Recurrent injury and the failure to comply with rehabilitation programs are not complications in the strict sense, but may indeed compromise the therapeutic effort. However, the development of postoperative infection or reflex sympathetic dystrophy, the loss of fracture reduction or fixation, and the failure of sutures are complications with potentially serious consequences. Precautionary measures are obvious and well-known, but it is worth emphasizing the advantage of soliciting the patient's commitment and cooperation postoperatively to avoid such occurrences. Although skin portals usually heal rapidly, they should be kept sterile and protected from contamination for at least 3 or 4 days. These seemingly innocuous portals often belie the magnitude of surgery performed within the joint under arthroscopic control. This is to the patient's advantage, but they must recognize that intraarticular procedures usually recover more slowly than the overlying skin, and that temporary modification of activities for protection or rehabilitation is of considerable importance.

BIBLIOGRAPHY

Committee on Complications, Arthroscopy Association of North America. Complications in arthroscopy: the knee and other joints. Arthroscopy 1986;2(4):253.

Cope R. The surgery of the rheumatoid wrist: postoperative appearances and complications of the more common procedures. Skeletal Radiol 1989;17(8):576.

Hastings DE, Silver RL. Intercarpal arthrodesis in the management of chronic carpal instability after trauma. J Hand Surg [Am] 1984;9(6):834.

Light TR. Salvage of intraarticular malunions of the hand and wrist: the role of realignment osteotomy. Clin Orthop 1987;214:130.

Whipple TL. Precautions for arthroscopy of the wrist. Arthroscopy 1990;6(1):3.

Zemel NP. The prevention and treatment of complications from fractures of the distal radius and ulna. Hand Clin 1987;3(1):1.

14

Postoperative Management and Rehabilitation

*T*he principal advantage of minimally invasive surgical procedures is that postoperative morbidity due to surgical exposure is reduced. Using methods of access such as arthroscopy or stereotaxis to reach internal lesions does not compound the injury with additional surgical trauma. To incise a ligament to repair another ligament is somewhat counterproductive. If conventional surgical access to remote anatomic regions is too arduous, the treatment may be worse than the original problem. But if internal lesions can be reached and removed or repaired with minimal incisional trauma, the indications for definitive surgical treatment can be relaxed and early intervention becomes plausible.

Arthroscopy has tipped the balance of risk versus benefit for many disorders of the wrist, as it has for other joints. Postoperative management is focused on the offending pathology. Following diagnostic arthroscopy of the wrist, recuperation entails only a concern for the portals. A sterile compressive dressing should be applied for 3 to 5 days until the portals are sealed and dry to protect the joint from contamination (Fig. 14-1). The dorsal wrist capsule is superficial, and bacteria in a moist skin puncture can easily find its way to the joint. Mobility, however, need not be restricted unless instruments are repeatedly inserted into the joint. In this case, a volar splint can be incorporated into the bandage for 5 to 7 days to hold the wrist extended while the capsule punctures seal.

Other postoperative considerations depend on the pathology encountered and the treatment rendered. Excision of portions of synovium, cartilage, or bone require little postoperative protection. Arthroscopic ganglionectomy, excision of a torn triangular fibrocartilage (TFC), and removal of osteophytes or loose bodies all can be followed by immediate mobilization. These procedures require no extensive recuperation or protection. The patient's comfort can guide the return to function.

More extensive arthroscopic synovectomy should be splinted until bleeding from areas of resection is unlikely. After 4 or 5 days, mobilization can safely begin. Arthroscopically reduced fractures, repaired ligaments, or cartilage reattachment requires the same healing time as repair by open techniques. These problems still demand immobilization; however, there

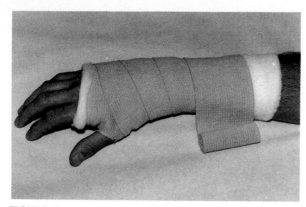

FIGURE 14—1.
A soft postoperative wrist dressing.

is no concern for adhesions to incisional scars when there are no incisions, and there is much less risk of reflex dystrophy, trauma, and pain.

Rehabilitation is more difficult after prolonged immobilization of the hand. Efforts to mobilize early and return the patient to function or at least to activities of daily living as soon as practical are important. These concerns are lessened following minimally invasive surgery techniques compared to conventional incisions.

Still, circumstances may require the occasional services of a hand therapist. This assistance is invaluable when swelling or stiffness occurs, or when a patient's pain threshold is unusually low. In most cases, however, patients regain functional use of the wrist and require less postoperative supervision following arthroscopic procedures than they do after open procedures.

BIBLIOGRAPHY

Budka M. Elbow and wrist arthroscopy: perioperative nursing care. Orthop Nurs 1986;5(4):29.

Carlson JD, Trombly CA. The effect of wrist immobilization on performance of the Jebsen hand function test. Am J Occup Ther 1983;37(3):167.

Chamberlain MA, Ellis M, Hughes D. Joint protection. Clin Rheum Dis 1984;10(3):727.

Kaukonen JP, Karaharu EO, Porras M, Luthje P, Jakobsson A. The functional recovery after fractures of the distal forearm: analysis of radiographic and other factors affecting the outcome. Ann Chir Gynaecol 1988; 77(1):27.

Pryce JC. The wrist position between neutral and ulnar deviation that facilitates the maximum power grip strength. J Biomech 1980;13(6):505.

Index

ISBN 0-397-51023-3

90000